T0262042

Aphorisms
&
Quotations
for the Surgeon

Edited by
Moshe Schein MD FACS FCS (SA)

Professor of Surgery,
Weill Medical College of Cornell University
Attending Surgeon, Bronx Hospital Center, New York

tfm Publishing Limited
Castle Hill Barns
Harley
Shrewsbury
SY5 6LX
UK

Tel: +44 (0)1952 510061
Fax: +44 (0)1952 510192
E-mail: nikki@tfmpublishing.com
Web site: www.tfmpublishing.com

Design and layout: Nikki Bramhill
Cartoons: Barry Foley

First Edition   © 2003
Reprinted April 2005, 2009 and 2018

ISBN 978 1 903378 11 3

Neither the authors, the editors nor the publisher can accept responsibility for any injury or damage to persons or property occasioned through the implementation of any ideas or use of any product described herein. Neither can they accept any responsibility for errors, omissions or misrepresentations, howsoever caused.

Whilst every care is taken by the authors, the editors and the publisher to ensure that all information and data in this book are as accurate as possible at the time of going to press, it is recommended that readers seek independent verification of advice on drug or other product usage, surgical techniques and clinical processes prior to their use.

Printed by Gutenberg Press Ltd., Gudja Road, Tarxien, PLA 19, Malta.

Tel: +356 21897037; Fax: +356 21800069.

Dedication

Professor JR Farndon

1946-2002

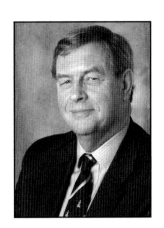

I first met John Farndon in 1989 when we were both introduced into the inner workings of the *British Journal of Surgery* (*BJS*) as associate (and very "green") editors. Over the years we rose together through the Journal's ranks - a period during which I came to realise what hard work was - through watching John. He was a hands-on editor, not a dilettante or a remote figurehead. He was endlessly painstaking and brought a very high degree of probity to his publishing work. A great interest lay in helping younger surgeons to write wisely and well; conversely, he was fierce with those who sought to deceive by duplicate or salami publication, or by false data and signatures. Outside the *BJS* he edited inter alia "A surgeon's guide to writing and publishing" with his friends Moshe Schein and Abe Fingerhut.

As joint editors from 1997, John and I enjoyed some success with the *BJS* impact factor and this, I believe, is largely due to John's diligence in seeking out only the best papers for publication, and detecting flaws where other more superficial assessors would have failed. Often such driven individuals are hard to work with, but not John. He was a big man not only physically and intellectually, but also in character - a generous and gentle person, with a whimsical sense of humour.

It was a great personal shock when I heard of his sudden death on 6 February 2002, not least because he had looked so well and had been in such excellent spirits when we had dinner together the previous evening. The days and weeks that followed this most unexpected of myocardial tragedies were distinguished by conversations with, and letters from, colleagues who had known my co-editor. It was abundantly clear that John Farndon had had a finger in so many local, national and international surgical pies that his passing would leave a great professional void. He will be greatly missed by so many of us - certainly as a colleague, but even more so as a friend.

John A Murie MA BSc MD FRCSEd FRCSG
Editor in Chief, British Journal of Surgery
Consultant Vascular Surgeon & Honorary Senior Lecturer,
Royal Infirmary of Edinburgh, Edinburgh, UK.

I was very lucky in my career as a publisher to work with Professor Farndon during his short lifetime. Indeed it was an honour to work with him on his last book entitled "A surgeon's guide to writing and publishing" which continues to sell well. I know he was pleased about that! On telling him about orders from all over the world, even some very remote parts, he always joked that it was one of his "aunties" who felt sorry for him! It was during this time that I got to know this incredibly intelligent, self-effacing, proud and professional person who had the most wicked sense of humour. At times of hair-pulling in the whole publishing process, he had this knack of diffusing any tension with his wry sense of fun. He encouraged my work in a kind and mentoring way, saying that I should "aim for the moon if I wanted to reach the stars". I will try my very best but on the way he will be missed.

Nikki Bramhill BSc(Hons) DipLaw Solicitor
Director - tfm publishing Ltd.

Only a few months ago John agreed to contribute to this book and then suddenly he vanished from the map and already he's sorely missed. John had a permanent smirk on his face, kind of a very subtle half smile - under a pair of bright and penetrating eyes. One had to meet with him only once or twice to be charmed - to fall in his net. As the Editor of the *BJS* John was a great friend to the international surgical community and admired around the world. The subtle combination of scholarly greatness and surgical leadership - wrapped in self-depreciation, genuine modesty and an immense sense of humour was the hallmark of his personality. In one of his last emails he wrote to me: "apologies for the delay in reply but have just returned from a late summer holiday - complete with knotted handkerchief and rolled up trousers!"

I know that John would have enjoyed this book and I dedicate it to his memory.

Moshe Schein MD FACS FCS (SA)
Professor of Surgery, Weill Medical College of Cornell University
Attending Surgeon, Bronx Hospital Center, New York

Contents

Foreword

Show me your favorite aphorism and I will tell you - who you are.
Karl H Bauer, 1890-1978

A good surgical aphorism makes me laugh or cry, for real aphorisms come directly from the heart! It conveys in a sentence or two what has been learned and experienced for many years.

I first became interested in surgical aphorisms during my training. Many aphorisms have been good friends to me, providing valuable advice in times of trouble; others I enjoyed for their insight and intellectual brilliance. Later I started sharing them with my residents. I have practised surgery in three continents, in vastly different surgical cultures but noticed that while each has its own set of aphorisms, the surgical truths remain the same.

According to Howard Fabing:
Since the days of Hippocrates, our father, the aphorism
has been the literary vehicle of the doctor ... laymen have
stolen the trick from time to time, but the aphorism remains
the undisputed contribution of the doctor to literature.

The term aphorism (aphorismos in Greek) denotes a "short, pithy sentence" or a "concise statement of a principle" or "a terse and ingenious formulation of a truth or sentiment". Clearly also rules and quotations may easily fall under such a description.

This book brings together a medley of over 1500 aphorisms, quotations, and rules by surgeons and non-surgeons, about surgery, surgeons and anything which may be relevant to the practice of surgery. In selecting these entries I was guided by Lewis Galantiére: "a truly serviceable book of quotations is not an expression of its compiler's preferences". Thus, I attempted to gratify all potential tastes by including ancient as well as contemporary entries, formal and colloquial, pronounced by surgical giants or anonymous, only guided by the prerequisite that the entry appeals to the surgical soul. I attempted however to eliminate self-congratulatory and self-righteous clichés commonly uttered by surgeons who stand up to speak in public. And, I used my editorial prerogative to bring a few of my own aphorisms, or what I think are mine, at the end of selected chapters.

My purpose was to provide the surgical reader with a source of large and widely varied surgical aphorisms and quotations. Most readers will probably use this book to decorate their lectures or manuscripts with relevant smart or entertaining entries. I hope however that this book will be simply read or browsed for pleasure: you will enjoy many of the entries, you will hate the others, and you'll discover that surgical truth is old, that what you think is a novel idea has been said before, that what you see around you was seen many years ago. It may contribute to your humanity and humility, perhaps even add maturity to your surgical personality and practice, and with a bit of luck increase your sense of surgical humor. Listen to Winston Churchill who said: "it is a good thing for an uneducated man to read books of quotations".

Moshe Schein
New York City
2002

Sources

My works are almost all aphorisms created in a short moment.
It is right, therefore, that my work soon will be forgotten. However,
I find solace in the knowledge that I have been one of the
best in my specialty in my time.
Vinzenz von Czerny, 1842-1916

Aphorisms are an integral part of our professional life as surgeons. We first hear them from our teachers during training, typically when things are not going so well in the operating room, or during rounds. We hear them from colleagues, and we adopt them and later use them in our own practice and research. In fact, aphorisms are also part of the surgical culture of every institution. There are those aphorisms that are home-made, some that are imported from others, and many that remain nameless and unidentified but still provide a valuable advice or insight, a collective wisdom for surgeons wherever they are.

I compiled the entries for this book from multiple sources: general books of familiar quotations, out-of-print books of medical quotations, small books of medical and surgical rules, books of medical and surgical history, surgical biographies, surgical journals, presidential addresses and the internet.

When known, the names of those who allegedly coined the entry is provided; when unknown it is not. It is obvious that many aphorisms and quotations simply float around, re-paraphrased in many versions, often claiming originality and under multiple authors. In order to provide historical perspective we have added the date of birth and death if known, of the authors. Authors cited without an accompanying date are hopefully still alive. Clearly, these entries belong to the collective surgical folklore, thus the property of the eternal surgical community and not deserving a copyright.

I have to admit that unfortunately this book is biased towards English language entries. It is however, extremely difficult to compile aphorisms and quotations which were never translated to English. We did attempt to gather entries among our Spanish, Russian and German-speaking friends, with disappointing results.

Readers who wish to comment or to add entries to the next edition of this book please e-mail me directly: mschein1@mindspring.com.

A comprehensive list of all sources used is impractical since only one or two entries were retrieved from most. Thus, the list below represents sources of more than a few entries, and could also serve as a recommended bibliography.

1. Golden Rules of Surgery. Augustus Charles Bernays. The CV Mosby Medical Book Co. 1906.
2. The Early Diagnosis of the Acute Abdomen. Zachary Cope. Oxford University Press. 1921.
3. History of Medicine. Fielding H Garrison. WB Saunders Company. 1929.
4. Surgeons All. Harvey Graham. Rich & Cowan. 1939.
5. Surgical Errors and Safeguards. Max Thorek. JB Lippincott Company. 1943.
6. A Surgeon's World. Max Thorek. JB Lippincott Company. 1943.
7. The Trials and Triumphs of The Surgeon. J Chambers da Costa. Dorrance & Company. 1944.
8. Surgery: Orthodox and Heterodox. William Heneage Ogilvie. Blackwell Scientific Publications. 1948.
9. Osler Aphorisms. Robert B Bean, Henry Schuman, Inc. 1950.
10. No Miracles Among Friends. William Heneage Ogilvie. Max Parrish. 1959.
11. Great ideas on the History of Surgery. Leo M Zimmerman & Ilza Veith. The Wiliams Wilkins Company. 1961.
12. Familiar Medical Quotations. Maurice B Strauss (Editor). Little Brown and Company. 1968.
13. Surgical aphorisms. Mark M Ravitch. Medical Times 1993; 101: 155-157.
14. The Gates of memory. Geoffrey Keynes. Oxford University Press. 1983.
15. Reflections. Alexander J Walt. Wane State University Press. 1999.
16. Aphorismen und Zitate fur Chirürgen. KH Bauer. Springer Verlag. 1972.
17. A Chance to Cut is a Chance to Cure. Rip Pfeiffer, Jr. Self Published. 1981.
18. Bailey and Bishop's Notable Names in Medicine and Surgery. Revised by Harold Ellis. 4th Edition. HK Lewis & Co, Ltd, London, 1983.
19. A little Book of Doctors Rules. Clifton K Meador. Henry & Belfus, Inc. 1992.
20. A Miracle & a Privilege. Francis D Moore. Joseph Henry Press. 1995.
21. Aphorisms. Charles H Mayo & William Mayo. Mayo Foundation. 1977.

22. A surgeon's little instruction book. Daniel J Waters. Quality Medical Publishing, Inc. 1998.
23. Surgery. An Illustrative History. Ira M. Rutkow. Mosby. 1993.
24. Surgical reflections. Seymour I Schwartz & Joe Wilder. Quality Medical Publishing, Inc. 1993.
25. Surgical Reminiscences. Claude H Organ (Editor). Archives of Surgery. 2001.

Acknowledgements

A large number of surgical friends and colleagues around the world provided aphorisms and sources. Many are cited along their contributions. The following deserve special acknowledgement (in alphabetic order).

Denis M Arkhipov, Moscow, Russia
Stephen Clifforth, Hamilton, Australia
Michael Dahn, Kansas City, USA
George Decker, Johannesburg, South Africa
Hernán Diaz, Santiago, Chile
Douglas Geehan, Kansas City, USA
Jerry Gerard, USA
Julian Losanoff, USA
Angus Maciver, Stratford, Ontario, Canada
Thomas Matthews Haizlip Jr., Linville, North Carolina
PO Nyström, Linkpoing, Sweden
Eric Olivero, San Francisco de Macorís, Dominican Republic
Ramesh Palagugu, Brooklyn, USA
Youry Vladimirovitch Plotnicov, St. Petersburg, Russia
Paul Rogers, Glasgow, Scotland
Avi Roy-Shapira, Israel
Sai Sajja, Bronx, New York
Ulrich Schöffel, Freiburg, Germany
Alfredo Sepúlveda, Santiago, Chile
Boris Shavchuk, Moscow, Russia
Panduranga Reddy Yenumula, Bronx, New York

Special thanks to all members of SURGINET (an international surgical forum on the internet) for their ongoing input and stimulation.

Introduction

Aphorisms - pithy bites of memorable prose - are a part of the culture of medicine. They are collected, as quotations, metaphors and even parables, because they form a store of knowledge and a kind of history of ourselves. Aphorisms are also an effective mechanism to communicate the complexities of the received wisdom of our profession from teacher to pupil in a brief and easily remembered form.

Such epitomes were more widely used in that not so distant time past when medical education, as well as consultation between physicians, was conducted at a more leisurely pace and within a more intellectual framework than usually characterizes these activities today. The once prominent pedagogic position of aphorisms seems to me to have faded somewhat in current medical education, with its new emphasis on quantitative evidence. But, there is an important place for the wisdom contained in aphorisms, a wisdom that still needs to be apprehended by each succeeding generation of physicians. Apt aphorisms still need to be quoted. And, perhaps, apt new ones need to be generated.

Collections such as this book usually are consulted as a work of reference. The objective may be to find the exact phrase to make a teaching point more memorable, or to capture a bon mot that will trump a discussion or settle an argument, or to find a memory device for future personal recall. Books of aphorisms are also perused simply for the enjoyment of the reader, an activity in which the reader's views and prejudices are brought to bear not only in judging the aptness of a quoted statement but also in the enthusiasm with which the aphorism is greeted.

While most aphorisms with a medical focus are teaching epitomes, there are many others that are of more general content and interest. These can be more or less philosophical, or cautionary, or cynical, or all three qualities in various proportions. Here are some I consider to be apt and topical. First, along a somewhat philosophical note, this observation from the author, Cormac McCarthy:

> "In history there are no control groups.
> There is no one to tell us what might have been."

Then, this somewhat cynical but true statement, usually attributed to Winifred Castle but in some quarters to the Scots poet, Andrew Lang:

> "Researchers use statistics the way a drunkard uses a
> lamp post, more for support than illumination."

And, this cautionary remark about ourselves from Barnaby Rich:

> "The inexpert captain, and the unlearned physician, do
> buy their experience at too dear a rate, for it is still
> purchased with the price of men's lives."

Any collection of aphorisms and quotations necessarily is a reflection of the collector's view of the world. The items chosen for inclusion, as well as those rejected, embody elements of the tastes, hopes, fears, memories, politics and prejudices of the collector. Some of my world view is reflected in the quotations above. Some of Dr. Schein's weltanschauung, despite his prefatory disclaimer, is contained in the collection of aphorisms within the covers of this book. And you, the reader, will now add your vision as you peruse and consult this valuable volume.

Robert E Condon, MD, MSc, FACS
Professor and Chairman, Emeritus,
Department of Surgery
The Medical College of Wisconsin
Milwaukee, USA

Aphorisms

Defining a literary companion

ăph'orĭsm, n. Short pithy maxim. Hence or cogn. **ăph'orĭsm**ic, **ăph'orĭs**tic, [IST], aa., **ăph'orĭs**tically adv. [f. F *aphorisme, (obs.) aff-*, or med L f. Gk *aphorismos* definition, f. *aphorizó* (*horos* boundary), see -ISM]

The Concise Oxford Dictionary of Current English. The Oxford University Press, 1996.

Unlike the direct lexicographer (above), the philosophers have a different and useful ploy in definition. They identify those things which something is not, and that which remains is that which it is. So with aphorism: what of maxim, and the close relatives of dictum, axiom, truism, platitude? What of that tacky stepsister, the cliché? The medical obscurities of "prognostic criteria" and "levels of evidence" pale into relative insignificance at this trivial, semantic, intellectual challenge.

Looking at the problem through the lens of surgery, we deduce that a maxim is a general surgical truth ostensibly drawn from science. These are those things we learned as students or residents, and now disbelieve, or have forgotten. They were usually prefaced by "Always" or "Never!". A dictum is a pronouncement, most often by a so-called "expert", which in terms of levels of evidence we are told must score a clear, straight five at the bottom of the list. They are the considered statements made by Chairmen of Surgical Departments or Expert Surgical Committees. It is essential that these dicta are handed down with gravitas and restrained pomposity. An axiom is a self-evident truth, often cringingly obvious. Under the pantheon of "the sicker you are, the worse you do", we find, for example, the prognostic criteria for pancreatitis. A truism is also a type of self-evident truth, which seldom requires discussion. An example could be: a surgeon is someone who wants to do surgery; an anaesthetist is someone who doesn't want to give anaesthetics. A platitude is a commonplace remark, solemnly delivered, and here we have the proud aphorisms of others (people we dislike, or find shallow). This genre is stated, after due reflective pause, on ward rounds and at meetings by senior surgeons, and is characteristically mawkish.

That tacky stepsister, the cliché is a hackneyed statement, characteristically trite.

> Hush little bright line,
> Don't you cry,
> You'll be a cliché
> By and by.
>
> **Fred Allen**

In the surgical world the density of clichés increases as we levitate through the successive strata of administration and bureaucracy. In the rarefied stratosphere of higher administration we might find administrators solemnly attempting to "expand the envelope of surgical care, on a seamless platform at all of primary, secondary and tertiary levels, with all the delivery players coming to the party, and health care being accessible, affordable and available to all clients" (read "patients").

Now that we have cleared the linguistic playing field, we can put aside the scalpel of cynicism, and return to aphorisms. We now know what an aphorism is not. What an aphorism is, is the crystal left in the semantic crucible. It glitters with wit, profound insight, and brevity; it is a revelation to new understanding. Its logic is striking, and the imagery often memorable, and moving.

We are most grateful to Moshe Schein for this remarkable collection of surgical aphorisms. Amongst them you will find a generous sprinkling of all the variants listed above, and your identification and categorisation of them will, I suspect, be purely personal.

David M Dent
Professor and Chairman
Department of Surgery
Faculty of Health Sciences
University of Cape Town
Observatory 7925, SOUTH AFRICA

Surgical Aphorisms

As friends for the road

On the first day of my internship in 1984 I found myself scrubbed as third assistant on an abdominal aortic aneurysm repair. The surgeon was my Chairman, Raphie Adar, and my role was to hang on to a pair of heavy Deaver retractors. I did not see nor understand much of what was going on, but when suddenly a huge gush of blood flooded the operative field and everyone became really excited, I realized that something was going terribly wrong. I was visibly shaken. My Chairman reached into the area of bleeding (which turned out to be a nasty tear at the bifurcation of the inferior vena cava), and calmly regained control. Then, noticing my apprehension, he turned to me and said: "Asher, whenever you encounter massive bleeding, the first thing to remember is that it is not your blood". Needless to say, I have adopted this aphorism and it has served me well throughout my training and later in practice as a teacher of trauma surgery - often to the sound of audible bleeding.

For many of us, aphorisms and quotations become good friends for the professional road. This is because aphorisms are not merely links to our heritage or delightful insights into our profession. Much more importantly, they frequently offer practical advice that is immediately applicable to what we do inside and outside the operating room. A good aphorism often passes from generation to generation, guiding surgeons to a safe and sound course of action. I am often fascinated by the fact that a surgeon from the past whom I have never met (and sometimes never even heard of) can offer me so much wise advice when I am facing a dilemma or a difficulty. That such advice is relevant and applicable after a century or more fills me with huge admiration for colleagues from the past who faced the same dilemmas under much more adverse circumstances. With minimal technology and support but with much wisdom, prudence and keen observation they still won their battles - truly amazing professionals.

Last week I found myself trying to teach yet another mildly unenthusiastic resident the fine details of a safe single layer hand-sewn bowel anastomosis. After all, in the age of the stapler, a hand-sewn anastomosis is becoming sort of "not cool"... Halfway through the anastomosis I found myself quoting Doctor William Silen: "if it looks good, it might work. If it does not look good, it will never work". And it definitely did NOT look good. I have never even met Doctor Silen, but I heard this aphorism often when I myself was learning to suture bowel from my mentors who trained with him. Through this quotation Doctor Silen has reached out and taught my resident a really valuable lesson that will serve her well in her own career. Such is the power of the good aphorism.

Asher Hirshberg, MD
Associate Professor of Surgery
Michael E DeBakey Department of Surgery
Baylor College of Medicine
and Director of Vascular Surgery
Chief, Blue Surgery Service
Ben Taub General Hospital
Houston, Texas.

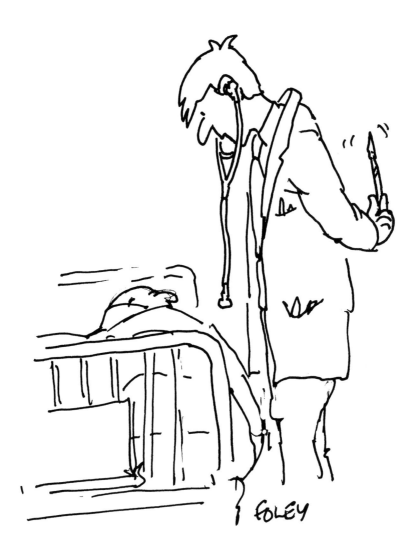

No incision signifies indecision, provided you can decide.

Chapter 1

Abdominal surgery

1   It is safer to look and see than to wait and see.

Sidney Cuthbert Wallace, ~1907

2   My experience in my first case emboldened me to use thermocautery and ligature of the larger vessels, and the excellent result justified my decision. In fact, after my experience with these three cases, I should hardly hesitate to attack almost any hepatic tumor without regard to its size.

William W Keen, 1837-1932

3   To open an abdomen and search for a lesion as lightly as one would open a bureau drawer to look for the laundry, may mean lack of mental overwork to the surgeon, but it means horror to the patient.

J Chalmers Da Costa, 1863-1933

4   The flat abdomen is a good abdomen.

George GA Decker

As long as the abdomen is open you control it. Once closed it controls you.

5   Abdominal closure: if it looks all right, it's too tight - if it looks too loose, it's all right.

Matt Oliver

6   At times it seems as though there is a brain in the suction tip that allows it to find the perfectly appropriate adhesion plane between bowel wall and parietal peritoneum.

Timothy Fabian

7   As long as the abdomen is open you control it. Once closed it controls you.

8   Every abdominal surgeon should have a gastric tube passed through his nose for 24 hours.

9   Never irrigate over a wider area than has been contaminated.

10   To prevent adhesions is to prevent wound healing.

11   Better to leave a piece of peritoneum on the bowel than a piece of bowel on the peritoneum.

From the editor

◆ The gut bursts out either because you did not close the tummy properly or it has no place inside.

◆ Dehiscence of the abdominal wound represents a spontaneous decompression of intra-abdominal hypertension.

◆ Abdominal closure: big continuous bites, with a monofilament and above all, avoiding tension; this is how to avoid dehiscence and herniation.

◆ A "planned hernia" is when you close the abdomen in such a way as to produce an incisional hernia, which you can then repair in a year or so.

◆ Anastomosis: the enemy of good is better; the first layer is the best - why spoil it?

Chapter 2

Academics

1   When you are certain of your knowledge
you need neither letter nor seal, for the work
praises the master.

Caspar Stromayr, 16th century

2   There is only one way to train capable
university teachers - one way that has been
practically tested - and that is to secure for
the universities the most distinguished men
of science, and to furnish them with the
necessary equipment for their teaching.

Theodor Billroth, 1829-1894

3   There is a lot of room at the top of the
profession, but it is a long, hard climb, and
there is no elevator running above the lower
floors. Some people wait for life for an
elevator to start, or take an attractive lift that
only goes part of the way. Others sit down
and complain and abuse all who toiled up
the stairs. Many things come to him who
waits, but seldom the thing he waits for.

J Chalmers Da Costa, 1863-1933

It is a simple system here: if you do not agree with the style or requirements of the man above you, you leave.

John C Goligher

1912-1998

4   The makeup of the ideal surgical professor: certainly it requires teaching ability. But, in addition to proficiency in the art and ability to teach, a professor must be one who is also trying to improve the science and art in which he works. We have seen enough of successful practitioners of medicine and surgery who have utilized their teaching positions to increase their practices and who, when they are gone, have left neither pupils, nor work which have furthered the advancement of the field in which they labored.

Elliot Carr Cutler, 1888-1947

5   The surest way to be a chair ... is to isolate oneself from teaching chores and become apprenticed to a scientist in a place such as the National Institute of Health where there are no medical students on whom one needs to waste one's precious climbing time.

Carl A Moyer, 1908-1970

6   In America there is some large gathering going on every week of the year, and the big men in surgery tend to attend about half of them. The same man who, in his hometown, rises at five and lies down at nine, becomes for a brief week a playboy, a cheerful companion, a retailer of delightfully humorous stories with a faintly blasphemous tinge. The meetings over, he and his fellows return, giant refreshed, to the main grim task of American surgery.

William Heneage Ogilvie, 1887-1971

7   I know admirable whole-time professors. I know none who would not be improved by private practice ... which would keep them human, for in it they would be dealing not with cases in a series but with human beings ... it would keep them humble, for their work would have to stand comparison with that of their colleagues.

William Heneage Ogilvie, 1887-1971

8   In Medicine there are many Popes but none faultless.

Karl H Bauer, 1890-1978

9   The Department of Surgery is like a boat at sea: I'm the captain and my responsibility is to steer. You are the oarsman; your responsibility is to furnish the power without rocking the boat too much.

Owen H Wangensteen, 1898-1981

10   Unless professors of surgery are actually capable surgeons, the whole structure of American surgery is threatened with collapse.

J Engelbert Dunphy, 1908-1981

11   It is a simple system here: if you do not agree with the style or requirements of the man above you, you leave.

John C Goligher, 1912-1998

12   Grand rounds: a well attended but occasionally esoteric gathering whose chief purpose some days seemed to be the glorification of the speaker rather than the transfer of knowledge from the haves to have-nots.

Jack Pickleman

13   Enough of the patronizing and gratuitous comments that are made at so many surgical meetings. Let the real debate begin!

Donald E Fry

From the editor

◆ The "Old Chairman Syndrome": at the lecture hall he preaches what he's heard at the last Association Meeting; on his own patients he practises what he did thirty years ago.

◆ How to advance rapidly in a modern surgical academic career? Publish more about less.

It is as much an intellectual exercise to tackle the problems of bellyache as to work on the human genome.

Chapter 3

Acute abdomen

1   Behold, my belly is as wine which hath no vent; it is ready to burst like new bottles.
Job, The Bible

2   It's this damned belly that gives a man his worst troubles.
Homer, 1050-850 BC

3   Pains occurring about the stomach, the more superficial they are, the more slight are they; and the less superficial, the more severe.
Hippocrates, 460-377 BC

4   When belly with bad pains doth swell, it matters nought what else goes well.
Saadi, 1184-1291

5   When in front of an acute abdomen, consider ectopic pregnancy, think always about it, thinking about it again is not enough, and still go on thinking about it.
Henri Mondor, 1885-1962

6   Two things surgeons fear the most are God and Peritonitis.
Henri Mondor, 1885-1962

7   There can be no question that in acute abdominal disease it is of the utmost importance to diagnose early.
Zachary Cope, 1881-1974

8   It is a curious but well-known fact that many who are taken with abdominal pain in the daytime endure till evening before they feel compelled to send for a doctor.
Zachary Cope, 1881-1974

9   The temptation is often very strong to temporize and "see how things are in the morning".
Zachary Cope, 1881-1974

10   The general rule can be laid down that the majority of severe abdominal pains which ensue in patients who have been previously fairly well, and which last as long as six hours, are caused by conditions of surgical import.
Zachary Cope, 1881-1974

11   Never give up in acute disease.
Mark M Ravitch, 1910-1989

12   We all bring to our work a sense of analytic thinking and it is as much an intellectual exercise to tackle the problems of bellyache as to work on the human genome.
Hugh Dudley

13   For the abdominal surgeon it is a familiar experience to sit, ready scrubbed and gowned, in a corner of the quiet theatre, with the clock pointing midnight.... In a few minutes the patient will be wheeled in and another emergency laparotomy will commence. This is the culmination of a process which began a few hours previously with the surgeon meeting with and examining the patient, reaching a diagnosis, and making a plan of action.
Peter F Jones

14   Severe, acute abdominal pain always requires a surgical consultation.

Clifton K Meador

15   A good surgeon evaluating acute abdominal pain is equivalent to a highly sensitive and specific laboratory test.

Clifton K Meador

16   An acute surgical abdomen is when a good surgeon says it is an acute surgical abdomen.

Clifton K Meador

17   There are two categories of emergent surgical patients: with peritonitis in the abdomen and with peritonitis in the head.

Denis M Arkhipov

18   Never let the skin stand between you and the diagnosis.

19   There are only three things needing immediate diagnosis in abdominal surgery: intestinal strangulation, peritonitis and a ruptured aneurysm.

From the editor

◆ This is what makes emergency abdominal surgery so exciting and demanding: the ever looming surprises and the anxiety about whether you are able, or not, to tackle it competently.

◆ The aim is to operate only when necessary but not to delay a necessary operation.

◆ You can shit on the peritoneum once and it will forgive you, but not a second time.

◆ Continuity of care is a "*sin qua non*" in the optimal care of the acute abdomen. Such patients need to be frequently re-assessed by the same clinician who should be a surgeon. But why should we be re-inventing the wheel? Why don't we learn? The place for the patient with acute abdominal conditions is on the surgical floor, surgical ICU, or in the OR and under the care of a surgeon - yourself! Do not shake off your responsibilities.

Chapter 4

Amputations

1   If the limb must be cut off, and nothing else will help, or if it has helped but the limb cannot be preserved, you should advise the patient to go to confession and receive the Holy Sacrament on the day before you amputate.

Hans von Gersdorff, 1480-1540

2   In the heat of fight, whether it be at sea or land, the chirurgeon ought to consider, at the first dressing, what possibility there is of preserving the wounded member; and accordingly, if there be no hope of saving it, to make his amputation at that instant, while the patient is free of fever.

Richard Wiseman, 1620-1676

3   A man will bear bleeding better after an amputation of the arm than the leg.

John Hunter, 1728-1793

Any fool can cut off a leg - it takes a surgeon to save it.

George G Ross

1834-1892

4   I have yet legs left and one arm. Tell the surgeon to make haste and get his instruments. I know I must lose my right arm and the sooner it is off the better.

Horatio Nelson, 1758-1805

5   Surgery will prescribe the amputation of limbs in extreme cases where this sacrifice is indispensable to the preservation of life.

Pierre-Francois Percy, 1754-1825

6   Any fool can cut off a leg - it takes a surgeon to save it.

George G Ross, 1834-1892

7   Amputation of a finger or toe is minor surgery, of the thigh is major. Who can draw the dividing line?

Augustus Charles Bernays, 1854-1907

8   War surgeons should try to emulate the dexterity of their ancestors, who had to perform amputations at lightning speed.

John Berry Haycraft, 1884-1941

9   If I refuse to allow my leg to be amputated, its mortification and my death may prove that I was wrong; but if I let the leg go, nobody can ever prove that it would not have mortified had I been obstinate. Operation is therefore the safe side for the surgeon as well as the lucrative side.

George Bernard Shaw, 1856-1950

10   Lose a leg rather than life.

Chapter 5

Anatomy

1 A blind man works on wood the same way as a surgeon on the body, when he's ignorant of anatomy.
   Guy de Chauliac, 1300-1368

2 Who are the men in the profession, that would persuade students that a little anatomy is enough for a physician, and a little more, too much for a surgeon? God help them!
   John Hunter, 1728-1793

3 An intimate knowledge of physiology is necessary to make a successful operator as is anatomy.
   Augustus Charles Bernays, 1854-1907

4 A bad anatomist can be a reckless butcher, but not an artistic surgeon.
   Augustus Charles Bernays, 1854-1907

A blind man works on wood the same way as a surgeon on the body, when he's ignorant of anatomy.

Guy de Chauliac, 1300-1368

5   The human body is the only machine for which there are no spare parts.

Hermann M Biggs, 1859-1923

6   It has been said that an anatomist never made a good surgeon, that it was the pathologist who made the surgeon.

William J Mayo, 1861-1939

7   The surgeon should not make beautiful anatomical preparations because he would destroy the natural arrangements.

August Bier, 1861-1949

8   In anatomy it is better to have learned and lost than never to have learned at all.

W Somerset Maugham, 1874-1965

9   The liver confounds the surgeon's dependence on anatomy.

J Foster

10   Who learns his anatomy only from books should operate on books only.

Chapter 6

Anesthesia

1   When, however, it becomes necessary to treat these patients by surgery we tie them to a table and have them held firmly in order that we may see exactly what we are doing.
Roland of Parma, ~1170

2   Three natural anesthetics: sleep, fainting, death.
Oliver Wendell Holmes, 1809-1894

3   The advent of anesthesia has made it so that any idiot can become a surgeon.
William Stewart Halsted, 1852-1922

4   The choice of an anesthetic is more often determined by the idiosyncrasy of the operator than by the necessity of the case.
Charles H Mayo, 1865-1939

5   Mr. Anesthetist, if the patient can keep awake, surely you can.
Wilfred Trotter, 1872-1939

General anaesthesia is like air travel: disasters usually occur during take off or landing.

Max M Simon

6   Nearly all drips set up at the start of an operation are not merely unnecessary, but harmful. At least half of the drips set up afterwards are an automatic routine or an assurance against worry, rather than a considered form of therapy.

William Heneage Ogilvie, 1887-1971

7   The causes of anaesthetic death are all too often mundane and obvious and rarely require much, if any, scientific investigations to establish them, provided a truthful account of the facts can be obtained.

Robert Macintosh, 1897-1989

8   All anesthetic agents are poisons - thus the fewer the number, the smaller the dose and the shorter the exposure, the better.

Mark M Ravitch, 1910-1989

9   What's blue & white anesthesia? The patient blue, the anesthetist white (blue and white are the colors of the Israeli flag).

Danny Rosin

10   A surgeon is someone who likes to operate; an anaesthetist is someone who doesn't like to give anaesthetics.

David M Dent

11   General anaesthesia is like air travel: disasters usually occur during take off or landing.

Max M Simon

12   The good surgeon deserves a good anesthesiologist, who is indispensable for the bad surgeon!

Oleg Zverev (From Russian - Youry Vladimirovitch Plotnicov)

13   Fifteen minutes spent preoperatively with a patient is worth 15 mg of morphine as a premedicant.

Stephen J Prevoznik

14   He is not even fit for a haircut under local anesthesia.

15   Blood brain barrier (BBB): the screen between the surgeons and anaesthetists.

16   There is an inverse relationship between a surgeon's ability and the frequency he asks for more muscle relaxant.

17   If you can feel a pulse, don't panic.

18   There is no such thing as a "little anesthesia".

19   The laryngoscope is a tool, not a weapon.

20   The patient who can't be intubated should be intubated.

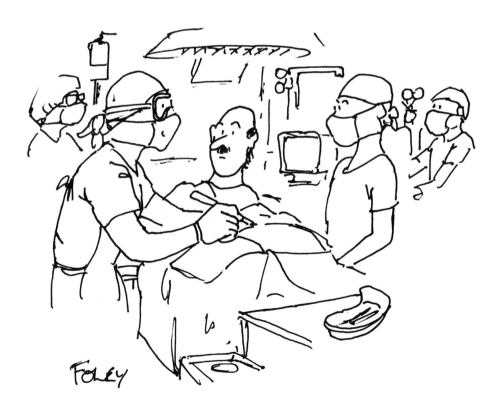

Mr. Anesthetist, if the patient can keep awake, surely you can.

Do not prescribe grantcillin and dinnercillin.

Moshe Schein

Chapter 7

Antibiotics

1   Patients can get well without antibiotics.
Mark M Ravitch, 1910-1989

2   Our arsenals for fighting off bacteria are so powerful ... that we're in more danger from them than from the invaders.
Lewis Thomas

From the editor

- Antibiotics for the fool is a tool which appears cool. But somebody pays the price as a rule.

- Start antibiotics prior to any emergency laparotomy; whether to continue administration after the operation depends on your findings. Know the target flora and use the cheapest and simplest regimen. The bacteria cannot be confused, nor should you be.

- Antibiotics in trauma: sooner and more is better than less and longer.

- No amount of post-operative antibiotics can compensate for intra-operative mishaps and faulty technique, or can abort post-operative suppuration necessitating drainage.

Chapter 8

Appendicitis

1 The point of greatest tenderness is, in the average adult, almost exactly 2 inches from the anterior iliac spine, on a line drawn from this process through the umbilicus.

Charles McBurney, 1845-1913

2 The mention of "expectant treatment" for appendicitis is to me like waving the banderillo's red scarf at el toro.

John B Murphy, 1857-1916

3 There are two kinds of appendicitis - acute appendicitis and appendicitis for revenue only.

Richard Clarke Cabot, 1868-1939

The appendix is generally attached to the cecum.

Mark M Ravitch, 1910-1989

4   In dealing with the stump of the appendix it is important to avoid two things: first, the simple ligation and amputation, leaving the mucosa membrane exposed, whether sterilized or not; second, a method that has been frequently practised, namely, that of ... burying the little stump by means of sero-serous sutures.

Howard Atwood Kelly, 1858-1943

5   The patient suffered from acute remunerative appendicitis.

Delbert H Nickson, 1890-1951

6   The experienced surgeon knows the pitfalls and dangers, which surround even the simplest operation. Perhaps he has himself lived through the sad experience of having a ligature slip when tying the appendiceal stump too short. He knows the dreadful penalty, which must follow ... if he ligates the appendiceal artery improperly.

Max Thorek, 1880-1960

7   The more educated is the layperson, the more experienced the surgeon, the prompter the intervention, the lower the toll of human life claimed by this treacherous enemy.

Max Thorek, 1880-1960

8   The appendix is generally attached to the cecum.

Mark M Ravitch, 1910-1989

9   The surgeon who can describe the extent of an appendiceal peritonitis has convicted himself of performing an improper operation.

Mark M Ravitch, 1910-1989

10   So I might have the immense privilege of relieving the pain, anguish, and threat to a wonderful small boy by making an incision in the right lower quadrant of his abdomen and taking out a pus-filled appendix skillfully and safely, my first operation ... I felt that this was both a miracle and a privilege. I still do.

Francis D Moore, 1913-2001

11   Beware drive through appendectomies.

Steven D Nishida

12   If she had appendicitis - she needed the operation. If she had PID - she deserved it.

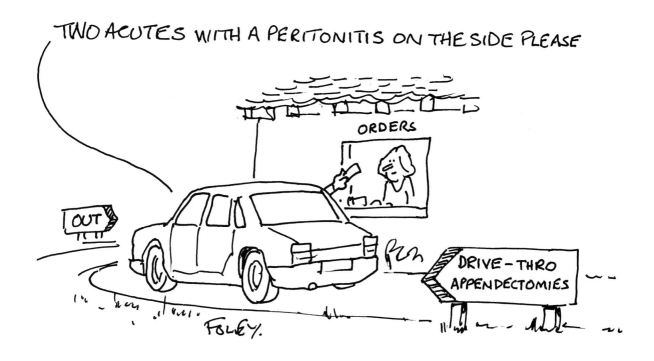

Beware drive through appendectomies.

From the editor

◆   We all know that whatever is the clinical presentation, whichever are the abdominal findings, always consider acute appendicitis at the back of your mind. However, there are two things in life that I will never understand: women and acute appendicitis.

Surgery should be

a merciful art; the

cleaner and

gentler the act of

operating, the less

the patient suffers.

Berkeley Moynihan,

1865-1936

Chapter 9

Art

1 And it should be the duty of physicians and surgeons to defend their art before the Courts, and not to permit further abuse of this art which is of so great importance.

Pierre Franco, 1500-1561

2 Chyrosurgery is an art, which teacheth the way by reason, how by the operation of the hand we may cure, prevent, and mitigate disease, which accidentally happen unto us.

Ambroise Paré, 1510-1590

3 Some call surgery a science, others an art; but in my opinion, it may claim either appellation.

Lorenz Heister, 1683-1758

4 Those therefore who estimate surgery by operation alone, and believe that nothing but long habit and practice is necessary to form the great surgeon, are grossly ignorant

of the art. We must think of the insolence and malevolence of those who represent it as a low mechanical art, which may be taught a butcher boy in a fortnight.

John Jones, 1729-1791

5   This last part of surgery, namely, operation, is reflection on the healing art; it is a tacit acknowledgment of the insufficiency of surgery. It is like an armed savage who attempts to get that by force, which a civilised man would get by stratagem.

John Hunter, 1728-1793

6   He who reduces the province of a surgeon to the performance of operations, and consequently directs his attention in a transient and careless manner to the less splendid parts of his profession, may learn the art of mutilating his fellow creatures, but will never deserve to be treated as a good surgeon.

John Pearson, 1758-1826

7   One should only advise surgery when there is a reasonable chance of success. To operate without having a chance means to prostitute the beautiful art and science of surgery.

Theodor Billroth, 1829-1894

8   The art of surgery is not yet perfect and advances now unimaginable are still to come. May you have the wisdom to live with them with grace and humanity.

William Stewart Halsted, 1852-1922

9   Surgery should be a merciful art; the cleaner and gentler the act of operating, the less the patient suffers.

Berkeley Moynihan, 1865-1936

10   As art surgery is incomparable to the beauty of its medium, in its supreme mastery required for its perfect accomplishment, and in the issues of life, suffering, and death, which it so powerfully controls.

Berkeley Moynihan, 1865-1936

11   The human body is a work of art and artistry is needed in dealing with its delicate tissues.

Berkeley Moynihan, 1865-1936

12   In the other fine arts, art is justified for the sake of art. In surgery it is a real need because upon the finesse and perfection of its artistry, the success of the surgical procedure largely and sometimes entirely depends. It is the art of the sculptor rendered with the heroism and skill of a lifesaver.

William D Haggard, 1872-1940

13   At the recent time ... surgery needs more men of the composer type.

Evarts Ambrose Graham, 1883-1957

14   Surgery is not a trade or art but a way of life.

Alexander A Artemiev

15   Surgery is not an art; it is a personality disorder.

From the editor

◆   You engage in danger, you take the risk, when the punishment for temporizing is greater than the peril of acting. This is why surgery is more an art, not only a science.

Chapter 10

Ascites

1   So he whose belly swells with dropsy, the more he drinks, the thirstier he grows.
Ovid, 43-17 BC

2   Those cases of empyema or dropsy which are treated by incision or the cautery, if the water or pus flow rapidly all at once, certainly prove fatal.
Hippocrates, 460-377 BC

3   The patient who looks like a yellow balloon needs a hepatic transplant.

So he whose belly swells with dropsy, the more he drinks, the thirstier he grows.

Ovid,

43-17, BC

In general the patient's ability to survive a major operation is inversely proportional to his productivity in society.

Chapter 11

Assessment

1 The glare in his eye and the strength of the grip.

2 The X-ray prognostic index: when the patient's X-ray folder is heavier than his or her body weight.

3 In general the patient's ability to survive a major operation is inversely proportional to his productivity in society.

4 Age/weight ratio: when > 1 it is bad news.

5 The undone, incomplete, unrepeated, physical assessment will get you, and the patient, into more trouble than any other problem.

Chapter 12

Assistants & Residents

1　Those about the patient must present the part to be operated upon as may seem proper, and they must hold the rest of the body steady, in silence, and listening to the commands of the operator.
Hippocrates, 460-377 BC

2　Have plenty of assistance, but not many assistants.
Augustus Charles Bernays, 1854-1907

3　A good assistant does not always make a good chief, but a bad assistant never does. A good chief has always been a good assistant.
Charles FM Saint, 1886-1973

4　I never fired any resident for a technical mistake, not even one who cut the common duct twice! I told him to stop racing the clock.
Warren H Cole, 1898-1991

Have plenty of assistance, but not many assistants.

Augustus Charles Bernays, 1854-1907

5   About common bile duct stones: those rocks are like residents; you never can find them when you're looking for them.

Robert M Zollinger, 1903-1992

6   The problem with your residents is that they have gland problems. If I could just get residents without glands I could get some work done.

Robert M Zollinger, 1903-1992

7   When practice in later years is too fast, and patient complaints are too obvious, and keeping up is too boring, and the wife has become too familiar, and the money too evanescent, and people have become less charming, even disgusting ... then the seeds planted in the residency will have borne their fruits.

H Grindinger

8   The more we choose residents, the more we get wrong.

Alvaro Sanabria

9   That resident has a direct neuron from the brain to anus.

Jose Di Sarli

10   A surgeon operates as good as his assistant permits.

11   The harder you pull - the more you learn.

12   High epididymal wedge pressure: common condition afflicting junior surgical residents.

13   The assistant should breathe at least four times a minute.

14   Tell your assistant how long the suture should be.

15   The surgical resident is like a mushroom: kept in the dark, fed shit, and expected to grow.

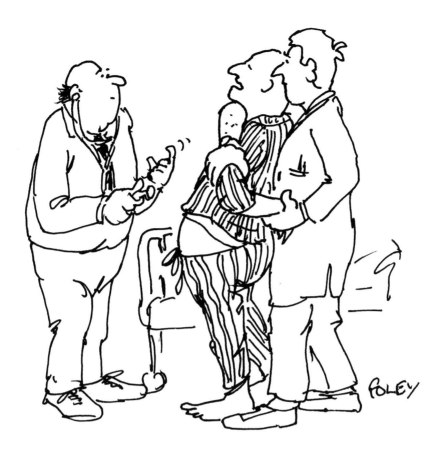

..... and they must hold the rest of the body steady,
in silence, and listening to the commands of the operator.

From the editor

◆ Poor surgeons can improve but poor assistants will never become good surgeons.

◆ On selecting surgical residents: good Lord I was thinking - are we choosing robots or human beings?

Cholecystectomy

should not be done

as a rule unless

the gallbladder is

diseased.

Augustus

Charles Bernays,

1854-1907

Chapter 13

Biliary

1   In cases of jaundice, it is a bad symptom when the liver becomes indurated.
Hippocrates, 460-377 BC

2   In dropsy of the gallbladder, in hydatid cysts of the liver and in gallstones we should not wait "til the patient's strength is exhausted", or "til the blood becomes poisoned with bile, producing hemorrhage"; we should make an early abdominal incision, ascertain the true nature of the disease, and then carry out the surgical treatment that necessities of the case demand.
James Marion Sims, 1813-1883

3   The gallbladder should be removed not because it contains stones, but because it forms them.
Carl Langenbuch, 1846-1901

4   Cholecystectomy should not be done as a rule unless the gallbladder is diseased.

Augustus Charles Bernays, 1854-1907

5   Gallstones are not so harmless as was formerly thought.

Augustus Charles Bernays, 1854-1907

6   If in the presence of jaundice the gallbladder is palpable, then the jaundice is unlikely to be due to stones.

Ludwig Courvoisier, 1843-1918

7   Jaundice is a disease that your friends diagnose.

William Osler, 1849-1919

From the editor

◆ When the gallbladder is "difficult" - go fundus down and stay near the wall.

The three biggest lies are "I will respect you in the morning", "the check is in the mail" and "it was dry when we closed".

Lee J Skandalakis

Chapter 14

Bleeding & Hemostasis

1 The blood is the life.
Deuteronomy, The Bible

2 It is a good plan in fresh wounds, except those in the abdomen, to allow a lot of blood to escape.
Hippocrates, 460-377 BC

3 When a surgeon finds himself in the presence of a wound, from which a great deal of blood is flowing, he should examine from which part it comes. If it flows from the wound by fits and spurts, then it is evident that it comes from an artery, and in that case it is limpid and of a lighter color. If the blood flows slowly, and is of a deeper color, it comes from the common veins which nourish the body.
Jean Yperman, 1260-1310

4 Hemorrhage can be stopped in four ways: by pressure exerted upon the vessel until the blood coagulates in the mouth of the

opening; by cooling of the part in which the wound is located; by actual or potential cautery; by ligature and torsion of the vein and artery.

Jean Yperman, 1260-1310

5   All bleeding eventually ceases.

Guy de Chauliac, 1300-1368

6   The physician today seems athirst for blood. Blood-letting, like wine-drinking, is right enough in moderation, but in excess, it leads to disaster.

Jean Fernel, 1506-1558

7   In letting blood three main circumstances are to be considered: who, how much, when.

Robert Burton, 1577-1640

8   Bleeding is the principal remedy in the cure of inflammatory disorders.

John Pringle, 1717-1782

9   Bleeding must be used with great caution when inflammation and fever run very high, lest the patient be reduced too much for the constitution to support life - for the very worst thing that could happen is the patient being reduced too low.

John Hunter, 1728-1793

10   The surgeon never suffers greater anxiety than when he is called upon to suppress a violent hemorrhage; and on no occasion is the reputation of his art so much at stake.

JFD Jones, ~1811

11   Blood is a very special juice.

Johann Wolfgang von Goethe, 1749-1832

12   The only weapon with which the unconscious patient can immediately retaliate upon the incompetent surgeon is hemorrhage.

William Stewart Halsted, 1852-1922

13 A French visitor to **Berkeley Moynihan (1865-1936)** after watching the latter's meticulous hemostasis: "is then your English blood so precious?"

14 We have at present many effective means of preventing blood clotting, but no means to accelerate clotting that do not bring the risk of spontaneous thrombosis in the cardiac and cerebral vessels ... can we not have some substance which when injected into the circulation ... seals cut vessels ... can we not have a hemostatic liquid that is sprayed on to the flap.

William Heneage Ogilvie, 1887-1971

15 Massive blood loss seals his fate. Do not wait ... operate.

Francis D Moore, 1913-2001

16 It's not bleeding until you can hear it bleeding.

Gail Waldby

17 Whenever you encounter massive bleeding, the first thing to remember is that it is not your blood.

Raphael Adar

18 The big thing is that nobody takes blood for granted anymore. We just don't get blood so easy, or give blood as easy, as before. Most folks want it that way, and I suspect they're right.

Edward Passaro, Jr.

19 To the surgeon the colors of winter and summer are red - the blood!

VA Zotov

20 There are 4 degrees of intra-operative hemorrhage: 1. "Why did I get involved in this operation?" 2. "Why did I become a surgeon?" 3. "Why did I study to become a doctor?" 4. "Why was I born?".

Alexander A Artemiev

21 The three biggest lies are "I will respect you in the morning", "the check is in the mail" and "it was dry when we closed".

Lee J Skandalakis

22   Blood bank is the surgeon's gas station.

23   The three words most often associated with re-operation for hemorrhage are: "it will stop".

24   You have to ligate the artery if the tip of the diathermy fits into its end.

25   One man's haemorrhage is another man's ooze.

26   Patients bleed whole blood - not components.

27   The most common cause of post-operative coagulopathy: poor hemostasis.

28   Operative atlases never bleed.

29   It is not the blood loss you can see that will get you, it's the blood loss you can't see.

From the editor

◆ The actively bleeding patient is like a bottomless bucket - you can't fill him.

◆ The most important clotting factor is the surgeon.

Breast cancer is a heterogeneous, systemic disease involving a complexity of host-tumor inter-relationships; variations in local-regional therapy are unlikely to affect survival substantially.

Bernard Fisher

Chapter 15

Breast

1   The cautery is used at first in order to prevent bleeding, but also because it helps to destroy the remains of the diseased tissues. When the burning is deep, prognosis is much better. Even in cases where indurated tumours of the breast occur that might be removed without danger of bleeding, it is better to use cautery, though the amputation of such a portion down to the healthy parts may suffice.

Aetius of Amida, 502-575

2   When cancer possesses the breast, it often causes inflammation of the armholes and sends the swellings even to the glandules thereof.

Ambroise Paré, 1510-1590

3   Even when a small portion of the breast is diseased, the whole mamma should be removed. The axillary glands should be dissected out by opening the armpit, but as much skin as possible should be preserved. I have done this since 1772. The older surgeons took away the skin and left the glands.

Benjamin Bell, 1749-1806

4   The early period of the complaint is beyond all doubt the most favorable period for extirpating it ... patients can be seldom convinced that there is any necessity for an operation while the disease continues in a mild state.

Henry Feardon, 18th century

5   The glands do not participate in the disease unless the system is strongly disposed to it and consequently their removal, however freely and effectually executed, cannot prevent the patient's relapse.

James Syme, 1799-1870

6   Why should we shave the under surface of the cancer ... the pectoralis major muscle, entire or all except its clavicular portion, should be excised in every case of cancer of the breast.

William Stewart Halsted, 1852-1922

7   The surgeon who removes a breast with a malignant tumor should be the mortal enemy of the one who will be closing the wound.

William Stewart Halsted, 1852-1922

8   I have drawn the impression that in dealing with mammary cancer surgery meets with more peculiar difficulties and uncertainties than with almost any other form of the disease.

James Ewing, 1866-1943

9   The main desideratum in the treatment of carcinoma of the breast as in other forms of cancer remains the discovery of some agent which will deal with the deposits outside the field of local treatment.

David H Patey, 1899-1977

10   I am not an experienced breast surgeon, but I have been interested in the aggressive therapy of cancer. I believe that our only hope is for the surgeon to be more aggressive ... I submit that one of the weaknesses of the present so called Halsted operation is our inability to get cancer out of the brachial plexus.

Owen H Wangensteen, 1898-1981

11   At the same time it is clear that there is a stage in every case of carcinoma of the breast during which the disease is a local lesion and therefore any form of local treatment must depend for its success on early diagnosis.

Geoffrey Keynes, 1887-1982

12   I had initiated an important advance in practice by trying to eliminate what I regarded as surgical malpractice - the performance of a grossly mutilating and illogical operation, when similar or slightly better results could be obtained by conservative surgery supplemented by radiotherapy.

Geoffrey Keynes, 1887-1982

13   The female psychologically identifies with the breast, which represents her narcissistic and sexual reality and also her relationship with others and with culture.

Dominique Gross

14   Breast cancer is a heterogeneous, systemic disease involving a complexity of host-tumor inter-relationships; variations in local-regional therapy are unlikely to affect survival substantially.

Bernard Fisher

From the editor

◆   There is a huge breast industry that feeds itself on the anxieties of breast cancer-prone women, and practises on scientific foundations which are no better than those which supported Halsted's radical mastectomy.

Chapter 16

Cancer surgery

1   The treatment of cancer is of two sorts: firstly that the affected part be radically and totally cut away with the entire disease by means of a very sharp knife ... the second type of treatment is palliative ...
William of Salicet, 1210-1277

2   The older a cancer is, the worse it is. And the more it is involved with muscles, veins and nutrifying arteries, the worse it is and the more difficult to treat.
Theodoric, 1205-1296

3   About cancers of tongue and mouth: this is so great an evil, that the slightest suspicion of it occasions very great uneasiness.
William Heberden, 1710-1801

4   We want a cancer hospital on its own foundation ... the subject is too large and its interest too great to be lodged in a pavilion subsidiary to any other hospital.
James Marion Sims, 1813-1883

In the world of surgical oncology: Biology is King, Selection is Queen, Technical manoeuvre is the Prince.

Blake Cady

5   When thou findest a fatty growth in the neck, and findest it like an abscess of the flesh and soft to the fingers, then sayest thou: "he has a fatty growth on his neck. I will treat the disease with the knife, paying heed to the vessels".

George Ebers, 1837-1898, surgical papyrus

6   Tumors belong in formalin jars.

William Stewart Halsted, 1852-1922

7   I unhesitatingly make this statement for all cancers, that when a whole year has passed, and the most careful examination can detect neither a local recurrence nor swollen glands, nor any symptoms of internal disease, one may begin to hope that a permanent cure may be affected; but after two years usually, and after three years almost without exception, one may feel sure of the result.

William Stewart Halsted, 1852-1922

8   In men nine out of ten abdominal tumors are malignant; in women nine out of ten abdominal swellings are the pregnant uterus.

Rutherford Morrison, 1853-1939

9   While there are several chronic diseases more destructive to life than cancer none is more feared.

Charles H Mayo, 1865-1939

10   There is a tremendous literature on cancer, but what we know for sure about it can be printed on a calling card.

August Bier, 1861-1949

11   The extirpation of cancer is very much like the eradication of quack grass. You cannot do a complete and thorough job in one sitting. When the field is surveyed a few weeks after the initial effort, surviving quack grass sprouts can be seen here and there still. And so it is, too, in the lymph node positive cancer cases.

Owen H Wangensteen, 1898-1981

12   The application of ... super radical procedures for extensive cancer may be more judiciously applied if the operating surgeons were required to follow these patients personally regardless of the outcome.

J Engelbert Dunphy, 1908-1981

13   Now that it has proved possible to resect half of the brain, an entire lung, any endocrine organ, much of the liver, any part of the digestive or urinary tract, to include the upper hemithorax in a forequarter amputation and to amputate the lower half of the body, it can be comfortably asserted that extirpative surgery has reached its final limit.

Mark M Ravitch, 1910-1989

14   A chance to cut is a chance to cure, but with the cutting done, the surgeon's work may be far from complete.

Robert A Briller

15   In the world of surgical oncology: Biology is King, Selection is Queen, Technical manoeuvre is the Prince.

Blake Cady

Addendum: occasionally the Prince tries to usurp the throne; he almost always fails to overcome the powerful forces of the King and Queen.

Moshe Schein

16   The rumour is tumour. The answer is cancer.

Gail Waldby

17   The jihad against lymph node is over.

18   The tumour is like an abscess - some are small but cause illness and discomfort, others are big before they make the patient feel sick.

19   However superficial the lump feels to you; at surgery it is much deeper.

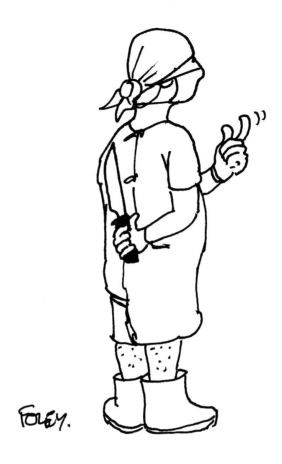

I will treat the disease with the knife.....

From the editor

◆ Technical wizardry can't overcome biological restraints.

◆ If a patient wants to go to Sloan Kettering Memorial Hospital, send him there.

Chapter 17

Circumcision

1   And ye shall circumcise the flesh of your foreskin; and it shall be a token of the covenant betwixt me and you.

The Bible

2   Circumcision is an ordinance for men, and honourable in women.

Mohammed

3   The Egyptians ... are the only people in the world who practise circumcision ... They practise circumcision for cleanliness sake - for they set cleanliness above seemliness.

Herodotus, 460 BC

4   My boss ... remarked, after I had performed a circumcision: "I can only hope the functional result will be better than the cosmetic!"

Edward Johnson Wayne, ~1960

Circumcision is perhaps the only operation which is done much better by non-surgeons.

Moshe Schein

He who farts -

lives.

Nicholas Senn,

1844-1908

Chapter 18

Colorectal

1   An abscess near the anus should not be left to burst by itself, but ... be boldly opened with a very sharp lancette, so that pus and the corrupt blood may go out. Or else ... the gut which is called rectum ... will burst ... for then may it ... be called fistula. And I have seen some who have seven or nine holes on one side of the buttocks ... none of which except one pierce the rectum.
John of Arderne, 1306-1390

2   He who farts - lives.
Nicholas Senn, 1844-1908

3   The examining physician often hesitates to make the necessary examination because it involves soiling the finger.
William J Mayo, 1861-1939

4   We suffer and die through the defects that arise in our sewerage and drainage systems.
William A Lane, 1856-1943

5   More surgeons' reputation is damaged by the bad result of a fistula than a laparotomy.

Lockhart-Mummerys, 1875-?

6   It is more important to insert the finger into the lower end than to put the thermometer into the upper end of the alimentary tract.

Zachary Cope, 1881-1974

7   Faecal incontinence after fistula is the result of aggressive surgeons, not progressive disease.

John Alexander-Williams

8   A good reliable set of bowels is worth more to a man than any quantity of brain.

9   Rectum: if you don't put your finger in it, you put your foot in it.

From the editor

◆ The only time human beings wish they could defecate and fart is when they are not able to do so.

◆ Colonoscopic perforation: the mechanism of the perforation determines the size of the hole, which should be thus managed selectively by the smart surgeon - not the blind gastroenterologist.

◆ In lower gastrointestinal bleeding, removing the wrong side of the colon is embarrassing. Removing any segment of the colon while the bleeding source is in the rectum is shameful.

◆ Think about acute diverticulitis as a left-sided acute appendicitis which is, however, usually treated without an operation.

Bringing a

colostomy out

through a

laparotomy

incision is like

putting a toilet in

the kitchen.

From the editor

Chapter 19

Colostomy

1   About colostomy: but it is surely far better to part with one of the conveniences of life, than to part with life itself. Beside, the excrements that are voided by this passage, are not altogether so offensive, as those that are voided per anum.
Lorenz Heister, 1683-1758

2   Of all the diseases to which man is liable, there is no one so inconvenient and disgusting as the artificial anus. How wretched is the patient from whom, despite his will, the alimentary, bilious and fecal matter contained in his intestines are constantly escaping.
Guillaume Dupuytren, 1777-1835

3   An artificial anus, it is true, is a grave infirmity, but is not insupportable.
Jean Zuléma Amussat, 1796-1856

◆   If you do a colostomy there will always be someone to tell you why not primary anastomosis; if you do a primary anastomosis there will always be someone to tell you why not colostomy.

Chapter 20

Complications

1 How many men in a year die through the timidity of those they consult for health!
Samuel Johnson, 1709-1784

2 Use the knife and the cautery to cure the intumescence and moral necrosis which you will feel in the posterior parietal region ... of self esteem ... after you have made a mistake in diagnosis.
William Osler, 1849-1919

3 We have our faults and our virtues; we meet with failures and achieve successes. Many of our faults are entirely unavoidable, and arise from the fact that medicine is not an exact science ... some things are quite impossible, and our work is carried out upon a living, breathing, complexity called a man, and not upon a jar, a chemical mixture in a retort, or a wooden Indian from the front of a cigar store.
J Chalmers Da Costa, 1863-1933

4 If you want a disaster of severe gravity - just try the wrong side or the wrong body cavity.
Francis D Moore, 1913-2001

How many men in a year die through the timidity of those they consult for health!

Samuel Johnson, 1709-1784

5   Surgeons may be blamed more than any other speciality for bad results, but then, they are admired, praised - even adored - for good ones.

Joan Cassell

6   Oh yeh, I forgot. None of us, of course, ever has any complication with whatever operation we perform. And if we do have complications they occur much less frequently anyway than those of others, and are never serious. And if they are serious, of course, they are not life threatening. And if they are life threatening, we never had a patient die from it. And if a patient does die from a complication it always is the resident who is the guilty person.

David Ligtenstein

7   Or if they die from the surgery, they would have died anyway without it, but the surgery improved their last few remaining minutes of life.

Gail Waldby

8   Search for a pneumonia in a wound.

Youry Vladimirovitch Plotnicov

9   This patient is FUBAR, which means: F***** Up Beyond Any Recognition.

Angus Maciver

10   If you create an albatross you live with it.

11   The one who does not operate does not have complications.

12   Everything in surgery is patient selection - the chief determinant of mortality and morbidity.

13   Always worry, worry, worry!

14   The source of most complications is in the operating room.

15   Good surgeons operate well; great surgeons know how to manage their own complications.

16   It is easier to stay out of trouble than to get out of it.

17   Do not congratulate yourself for saving a patient from a trouble inflicted by you.

18   More is missed by not looking than not knowing.

19   Minor complication is one that happens to somebody else.

20   If everything is going right you've done something wrong.

21   Surgical complications are more likely on public holidays.

22   Frequent dilemma: take your wife for dinner or the patient back to the OR?

23   Operating on doctors' families: a big compliment with most complications.

From the editor

◆ The number of iatrogenic diseases scattered around is approaching that of the natural ones.

◆ Somebody's leak is a curiosity - one's own leak is a calamity.

◆ The formula for Morbidity & Mortality in emergency surgery is simple: M&M= acute physiological status of the patient + underlying chronic status + magnitude of surgery.

◆ In surgery what is alleged to be a "piece of cake" may become a sponge cake saturated with blood.

Never operate on a patient who is getting rapidly better or rapidly worse.

Francis D Moore, 1913-2001

Chapter 21

Conservatism

1   He should refuse, as much as possible, difficult cures. He should never meddle with desperate cases.
Henri de Mondeville, 1260-1320

2   The surgeon, however, should leave the sick man alone rather than operate, if he is in any doubt: for it is safer to leave a man in the hands of his Creator, than to put trust in surgery or medicine concerning which there is any manner of doubt.
John of Mirfield, 14th century

3   Never, if you can help it, bereave a man of any part; for God's grace may be great upon it beyond the expectation of men.
Felix Wurtz, 1518-1574

4   Tis the chirurgeon's praise, and height of art, not to cut off, but cure the vicious part.
Robert Herrick, 1591-1674

5   It never can be right to counteract nature, and oblige her to do that she is not inclined to, and which she would otherwise accomplish better.

Percivall Pott, 1714-1788

6   When an operation is necessary think ten times about it, for too often when we decide upon an operation we sign the death warrant of the patient.

Charles Denonvilliers, 1808-1872

7   Let man learn to be honest and do the right thing or do nothing.

James Marion Sims, 1813-1883

8   It is less important to invent new operations and new techniques of operating than to find ways and means to avoid surgery.

Bernhard von Langenbeck, 1810-1887

9   Many times, when operating, the highest wisdom is to stop.

J Chalmers Da Costa, 1863-1933

10   When people have entered the seventies of their age, they usually find themselves growing conservative.

William J Mayo, 1861-1939

11   The surgeon whom I would select to tend my family must first know when not to cut, when and where to cut, how to cut, and when to stop cutting.

Charles W Mayo, 1865-1939

12   Allow patients to escape with the slightest attack of surgery your skill can supply.

Robert Tuttle Morris, 1857-1945

13   The greatest triumph of surgery today ... lies in finding ways for avoiding surgery.

Robert Tuttle Morris, 1857-1945

14   In surgery all operations are recorded as successful if the patient can be got out of the hospital or nursing home alive, though the subsequent history of the case may be such as would make an honest surgeon vow never to recommend or perform the operation again.

George Bernard Shaw, 1856-1950

15 The surgeon should always remember that operation is not synonymous with surgery, and that the primary object of surgery is not operation, but the cure of the patient.

Max Thorek, 1880-1960

16 It is greatly more to the surgeon's credit to avoid, than to perform an operation - to arrest the progress of pathology instead of operating to remove it.

Max Thorek, 1880-1960

17 Every hospital should have a plaque in the physicians' and students' entrances: "there are some patients who we cannot help; there are none whom we cannot harm".

Arthur L Bloomfield, 1888-1962

18 The mere withholding of an operation is not a virtue in itself.

Mark M Ravitch, 1910-1989

19 Too often, surgical therapy for elective conditions is postponed in elderly patients, in the hope, I presume, that the patient will die of some other disease before the present one threatens his life.

Warren H Cole, 1898-1991

20 Never operate on a patient who is getting rapidly better or rapidly worse.

Francis D Moore, 1913-2001

21 Doing something is sometimes worse than doing nothing.

Gail Waldby

22 The most difficult thing is to do nothing.

Norman M Rich

23 Surgery is always second best. If you can do something else, it's better.

John Kirklin

24 When the physician is at a loss, it is wiser to do nothing than to recommend what may be injurious.

David Craige

25   Time and Mother Nature are the surgeon's two greatest allies, and many a seemingly impossible situation can be converted to one that is merely a challenge by careful patience.

John Marshall

26   Do not mess around with mother nature.

Jonathan Meakins

27   Anything not worth doing is not worth doing well.

28   Don't fix nothing if it ain't broke.

29   Measure thrice, think twice, cut once.

30   A good retreat is better than a brave stand.

31   What some patients need is a little benevolent neglect.

32   It takes five years to learn when to operate and twenty years to learn when not to.

From the editor

◆ The fact that you do not know what to do does not mean that you have to do something.

The problem with calling in a consultant is that you may feel obliged to take his advice.

Mark M Ravitch,

1910-1989

Chapter 22

Consultation

1   When you are called to a patient if the matter appears to you too difficult ... do not be ashamed to send after one or two other surgeons so that they can help you and give you good advice from which you and the patient can derive great benefit: firstly, that you become aware that previously you have accomplished nothing or very little; secondly, whether you have neglected anything which is corrected by the others; thirdly, that you be aware if you left the wounded in a worsened condition; fourthly, if everything goes well, you will participate in the success. If things go wrong they will share the burden; fifthly, you will be praised by the sages who will then say: he desires to learn and neglects no one.

Hieronymus Brunschwig, 1450-1512

2   Also guard yourself, if an injury comes to you which you do not understand how to heal it, you should willingly direct him away to another, experienced master, so that

you may not ruin the person, as often happens with lesser Masters who through their neglect bring people from life to death.

Hans von Gersdorff, 1480-1540

3 Thou wilt also learn one necessary piece of humility, viz. not to trust too much on thy own judgement, especially in difficult cases; but to think fit to seek the advice of other physicians or chirurgeons.

Richard Wiseman, 1620-1676

4 The problem with calling in a consultant is that you may feel obliged to take his advice.

Mark M Ravitch, 1910-1989

5 If you cannot figure out a patient's problems perhaps someone else can.

Mark M Ravitch, 1910-1989

6 Seek consultation even if it is not sure to help; never be a lone wolf.

Francis D Moore, 1913-2001

7 "Surgical consult": like asking a barber if you need a haircut.

Eric Frykberg

From the editor

◆ Above all - avoid "consultantorrhea" which may adversely affect survival.

That child is

dying, and I wish

to God I'd never

been a surgeon.

Samuel Gross,

1805-1884

Chapter 23

Death

1   It sometimes occurs that the mouth is livid or black, the nostrils are pinched, and the eye deeper sunk than before; all these things are presages of impending death.
Pierre Franco, 1500-1561

2   Always give the patient hope, even when death seems at hand.
Ambroise Paré, 1510-1590

3   There's a sort of decency among the dead, a remarkable discretion: you never find them making any complaint against the doctor who killed them.
Molière, 1622-1673

4   Most men die of their remedies, not of their diseases.
Molière, 1622-1673

5   I prefer to die by the decree of God rather than by the hand of man.

Guillaume Dupuytren, 1777-1835

6   That child is dying, and I wish to God I'd never been a surgeon.

Samuel Gross, 1805-1884

7   We must celebrate ... today, my dear for on this day next year, I shall not be here.

Johan Mikulicz-Radecki, 1850-1905

8   Please stay with me for the night is falling. I have only another fortnight to live.

Johan Mikulicz-Radecki, 1850-1905

9   Before undergoing a surgical operation arrange your temporal affairs - you may live.

Remy de Gourmont, 1858-1915

10   It is said that the good die young. I am not sure of this, but I am quite sure that only the young die good. If the good do not die young, they will grow up to be as lonely as a moralist on the police force.

J Chalmers Da Costa, 1863-1933

11   There is only one ultimate and effectual preventive method for the maladies to which flesh is heir, and that is death.

Harvey Williams Cushing, 1869-1939

12   Above all, let us remember that our duty to our patients ends only with their death, and that in the preceding hours there is much that we can do for their comfort. At the very least, we can stand by them.

Alfred Worcester, 1855-1951

13   Deaths, for which I am inclined to think I am at fault, have occurred generally towards the end of many daily oophorectomies, when I may have been tired or possibly unclean.

John Homans, 1877-1954

14   I deeply regret I won't be able to see my own autopsy and find out what my left iliac artery looks like.

John Homans, 1877-1954

15   Every surgeon carries about him a little cemetery, in which from time to time he goes to pray, a cemetery of bitterness and regret, of which he seeks the reason for certain of his failures.

Rene Leriche, 1879-1955

16   The transition between life and death should be gentle in the winter of life. Death under these conditions, is invested with a certain grandeur and poetry, if it comes to a man when he has completed his mission ... There is nothing to fear, nothing to dread.

Rudolph Matas, 1860-1957

17   Patients are rarely afraid to die. They are always afraid if they are being deceived and seem to be abandoned. A good physician, a sympathetic surgeon clearly visible in the background, a united family, an attitude of aggressive optimism and a determination to control pain intelligently, can make these tribulations not only bearable but a deeply moving and ennobling experience.

J Engelbert Dunphy, 1908-1981

18   Every psychoneurotic ultimately dies of organic disease.

Mark M Ravitch, 1910-1989

19   Because the surgeon is so close to the reality of life in the balance and of death, he needs to develop skin of exactly the right thickness.

Francis D Moore, 1913-2001

20   All surgeons will at some point be part in a patient's unexpected death - all, without exception, at least once.

PO Nyström

21   Again and again I find that there are few things so quickly forgotten by the surgical system as a dead patient.

PO Nyström

22   Without reanimation there is no cremation.

Youry Vladimirovitch Plotnicov

23   Bleed him and purge him; if he dies, bury him.

24   Are we prolonging life or prolonging death?

25   If a pre-op patient tells you he's going to die - cancel the operation.

26   Surgeons' faults are covered with earth, and rich men's with money.

God gave you

ears, eyes, and

hands; use them

on the patient in

that order.

William Kelsey Fry,

1889-1963

Chapter 24

Diagnosis

1   All the causes of things cannot be seen, because they appear to depend on circumstances which are unknown, or appear to be accidental.

John Hunter, 1728-1793

2   We are too much accustomed to attribute to a single cause that which is the product of several, and the majority of our controversies come from that.

Justus von Liebig, 1803-1873

3   Diagnosis by intuition is a rapid method of reaching a wrong diagnosis.

J Chalmers Da Costa, 1863-1933

4   Surgeons ... ought to become the best diagnosticians; because the frequent use of exploratory incisions is a check upon diagnostic error.

J Chalmers Da Costa, 1863-1933

5   Beware of the diagnosis of hysteria, neurosis or neuralgia, unless organic disease can be excluded with certainty.

Rutherford Morrison, 1853-1939

6   Remember that exploratory incisions should not be made a cloak for diagnostic incompetence.

Rutherford Morrison, 1853-1939

7   Mistakes in surgical diagnosis occur not from want of knowledge but from carelessness, over-confidence, being in a hurry, or jumping to conclusions.

James Berry, 1860-1946

8   God gave you ears, eyes, and hands; use them on the patient in that order.

William Kelsey Fry, 1889-1963

9   The misleading symptoms are misleading only to one able to be mislead.

William Heneage Ogilvie, 1887-1971

10   A spot diagnosis is the surest way to a wrong conclusion.

Charles FM Saint, 1886-1973

11   Place your bets on uncommon manifestations of common conditions rather than on common manifestations of uncommon conditions.

Mark M Ravitch, 1910-1989

12   Diagnosis may be based on the X-ray or the tissue section, but not on the report.

Mark M Ravitch, 1910-1989

13   How does a surgeon measure the patient's pulse? Takes it for a second and multiplies by sixty.

Franz Bauer

14   Having lice doesn't mean not having fleas.

Jorge Bezama

15   When you hear hoof beats, think of horses, not zebras: common is common!

Gail Waldby

16   We diagnose that which we are thinking about, we think about that we know, and we know only that we have studied.

17   Treat the patient, not the X-ray.

18   The more the noise - the less the fact.

19   Fascinoma=something you don't see everyday.

20   Time is the greatest diagnostician.

From the editor ◆ The more non-indicated tests you order, the more false positive results are obtained, which in turn compel you to order more tests which lead to additional, potentially harmful, diagnostic and therapeutic interventions.

Chapter 25

Dogma

1   Our ancestors deserve our best thanks for the assistance which they have given us: where we find them to be right, we are obliged to embrace their opinions as truths; but implicit faith is not required from man to man; and our reverence for our predecessors must not prevent us from using our own judgments.

Percivall Pott, 1714-1788

2   The greater the ignorance, the greater the dogmatism.

William Osler, 1849-1919

3   It is now as it was then and as it may ever be; conceptions from the past blind us to facts which almost slap us in the face.

William Stewart Halsted, 1852-1922

4   He follows customs even when it is unreasonable or actually absurd. His headlight, like the glow of the glow worm, is

The greater the ignorance, the greater the dogmatism.

William Osler, 1849-1919

on the wrong end. He progresses but in a circle, like the hands of a clock. He is not the active man behind the gun, but the slow and often dull man behind the times. His ideas are from a reservoir and not from the spring.

J Chalmers Da Costa, 1863-1933

5   As the great Lord Bacon said, "much that was solid has sunk into the river of time, and much that was light has floated". Multiple assertions must not be taken as proof for books copy each other. A name does not prove a truth.

J Chalmers Da Costa, 1863-1933

6   We think so because all other people think so; or because we think we in fact think so; or because we were told to think so, and think we must think so.

Rudyard Kipling, 1865-1936

7   Failure to produce a scholarly environment for the embryonic surgeon will encourage unquestioning dogma that will be restrictive for future development.

William Silen

8   Sometimes these discussions confirm my first impressions of our species; it doesn't matter so much what you believe as long as you are dogmatic about it.

Charles Hendricks

Chapter 26

Drains

Drainage is a confession of imperfect surgery.

Howard Kelly,

1858-1943

1   When in doubt drain.
Robert Lawson Tait, 1845-1899

2   Drainage of the general peritoneal cavity is a physical and physiological impossibility.
JL Yates, ~1905

3   There are those who ardently advocate it, there are those who in great part reject it, there are those who, Laodicean-like, are lukewarm concerning it, and finally, some who, without convictions, are either for or against it ... as chance or whim, not logic may determine.
Joseph Price, 1853-1911

4   After draining the axillary abscess of Queen Victoria: "it occurred to me that in this deep and narrow incision, the lint, instead of serving as a drain, might have acted like a plug".
Joseph Lister, 1827-1912

5   The first and most important result of the war in the surgical world will be the abandonment once and for all of the drainage tube. Its day is past, and soon it will only be seen, where it should be, in the museum.

F Hathaway, ~1918

6   No drainage is better than the ignorant employment of it.

William Stewart Halsted, 1852-1922

7   A drain invariably produces some necrosis of the tissue with which it comes in contact, and enfeebles the power of resistance of the tissues toward organisms.

William Stewart Halsted, 1852-1922

8   Drainage of the peritoneum though one of the most important subjects in abdominal surgery, is yet one which stands in a most uncertain position.

Charles Bingham Penrose, 1862-1925

9   Drainage is a confession of imperfect surgery.

Howard Atwood Kelly, 1858-1943

10   Although more than five million surgical drains are used each year in the United States, their effectiveness, therapeutic indications, and efficiency remains an unsolved controversy.

JP Moss

11   If you have to use drains to take care of post-operative hemorrhage then you did not finish the operation.

◆ Despite the dictum that it is impossible to effectively drain the peritoneal cavity, drains are still commonly used and misused.

You can always give more, never less.

Chapter 27

Drugs

1   I firmly believe that if the entire *materia medica* as now used could be sunk to the bottom of the sea, it would be all the better for mankind - and all the worse for the fishes.

Oliver Wendell Holmes, 1809-1894

2   Tranquilizers have their major beneficial effects upon the staff, not the patient.

Mark M Ravitch, 1910-1989

3   Today surgeons and psychiatrists use drugs more than ever before. In their overuse and misuse lie many of the misfires of all medical care.

Francis D Moore, 1913-2001

4   If you do not know the exact dose of the IV drug: inject half the dose and slowly.

Ahmed Assalia

5   This dumb son of immigrant farmers who engendered in me a love for America doesn't understand how the Physician Leadership on National Drug Policy can continue to procrastinate in their moral and American obligation to promote complete and total legalization of street drugs.

Charles E Lucas

6   You can always give more, never less.

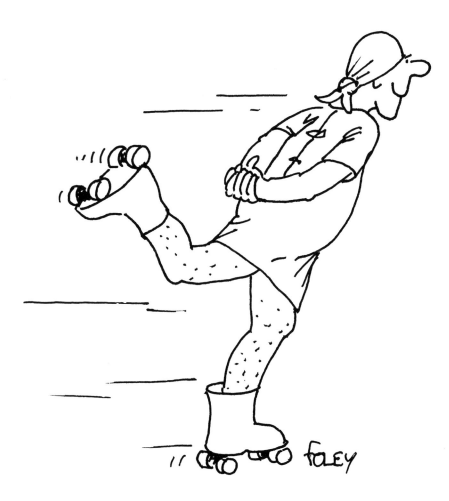

Tranquilizers have their major beneficial effects upon the staff, not the patient.

If the resident did

it badly, make him

re-do it; if he did

it badly again,

re-do it yourself.

Chapter 28

Education

1   It behooves practitioners of surgery to frequent the places where skilled surgeons operate, and to attend these operations diligently and commit them to memory.
Theodoric, 1205-1296

2   Thou shalt far more easily and happily attain to the knowledge of these things by long use and much exercise, than by much reading of books, or daily hearing of teachers. For speech how perspicuous and elegant so ever it be, cannot so vividly express any thing, as that which is subjected to the faithful eyes and hands.
Ambroise Paré, 1510-1590

3   I have thought it no disgrace to let the world see where I failed of success, that those that come after me may learn what to avoid; there being more instructiveness often in an unfortunate case than in a fortunate one.
Richard Wiseman, 1620-1676

4   What is most worth knowing, is soonest learned and least the subject of disputes.

William Cheselden, 1688-1752

5   Pointing out several cadavers: "these are the books your son will learn under my direction, the others are fit for very little".

John Hunter, 1728-1793

6   My lectures were highly esteemed, but I am of opinion my operations rather kept down my practice.

Astley Paston Cooper, 1768-1841

7   I never fail to impress on my students the great value of operations and vivisection on large dogs.

Augustus Charles Bernays, 1854-1907

8   You must always be students, learning and unlearning till your life's end, and if, gentlemen, you are not prepared to follow your profession in this spirit, I implore you to leave its ranks and betake yourself to some third-class trade.

Joseph Lister, 1827-1912

9   The education of a doctor which goes on after his degree is, after all, the most important part of his education.

John Shaw Billings, 1838-1913

10   According to Paget's figures, almost one third of any class of students made a mistake when they selected medicine for a profession. I am disposed to think that Paget's figures would apply today.

J Chalmers Da Costa, 1863-1933

11   Medical examinations: they are no tests of the man. They are only tests of his memory for facts. They tell us nothing of his judgment, tact, energy, enthusiasm, idealism, reason, observation, temperament, disposition, honesty, loyalty, courage, truthfulness, or intelligence. Memory of facts means little. The other things mean nearly all.

J Chalmers Da Costa, 1863-1933

12   Most medical students are attracted to surgery. Its positive results please them. The bloody drama of the operation fascinates them, the dramatic force of some great operator stirs their admiration. They hear little of failures. They know nothing of the haunting anxieties, the keen disappointments, the baffling perplexities, the dread responsibilities, and the numerous self-reproaches.

J Chalmers Da Costa, 1863-1933

13   We give too much attention to the development of memory and too little to developing the mind; we lay too much stress on acquiring knowledge and too little on the wise application of knowledge.

William J Mayo, 1861-1939

14   One of the signs of a truly educated people, and a broadly educated nation, is lack of prejudice.

Charles H Mayo, 1865-1939

15   Once you start studying medicine you never get through with it.

Charles H Mayo, 1865-1939

16   The safest thing for a patient is to be in the hands of a man engaged in teaching medicine. In order to be a teacher of medicine the doctor must always be a student.

Charles H Mayo, 1865-1939

17   The soldier is rewarded or promoted for risk of life and personal valor; an officer who is given authority to command the destruction of life may have spent but a few months in the training camp, while the medical officer who is responsible for the preservation of life devotes many years to preparation.

Charles H Mayo, 1865-1939

18   Reading papers is not the purpose of showing how much we know and what we are doing but is an opportunity to learn.

William J Mayo, 1861-1939

19   The best any of us can do as successful teachers of medical students is to instill principles, arouse interest, put the student on the right track, give him methods, show him how to study, and early to discern between essentials and unessential.

Harvey Williams Cushing, 1869-1939

20   Students should know which disorders should be treated by surgery and also know something of the dangers and complications of the surgical undertaking.

Elliot Carr Cutler, 1888-1947

21   Any arrangement which allows one's pupils to share completely one's daily work is the more stimulating and satisfactory method of exposition.

Elliot Carr Cutler, 1888-1947

22   In surgery most of our knowledge is based on what we learn from others.

William Heneage Ogilvie, 1887-1971

23   The worst thing that can happen to a young surgeon is that he should go immediately after taking his fellowship to a post where he has abundant practical work, but no time to read or to attend meetings, no time to think and write, and - still worse - no one to criticise or ask questions.

William Heneage Ogilvie, 1887-1971

24   But teaching is not simply talking, and often those who talk most, teach less. However, talking is necessary and silence... is by all means not always golden and a sign of depth and strength.

Charles FM Saint, 1886-1973

25   I have always believed, too, that the greater the teacher, the simpler his language... the greater the number of monosyllables the more readily is the subject matter understood.

Charles FM Saint, 1886-1973

26 Useful knowledge is meant to be applied. Useless knowledge may even be an encumbrance and may be occupying a cell that could be better employed.

Charles FM Saint, 1886-1973

27 It is a mistake to talk down to students, but rather to treat them as budding or potential equals - they prefer it - and their ego is satisfied.

Charles FM Saint, 1886-1973

28 Criticism is essential: if destructive, supply a remedy.

Charles FM Saint, 1886-1973

29 I failed in the primary Fellowship examination of the Royal College - I was ... inadequate in the ordeal of exposure to the savagely searching questions asked by experienced and sometimes rather alarming surgeons, who wanted to know how much a frightened young man could reproduce, from his only partially trained memory, of details of topographical anatomy, much of which had seemed to him to be of little or no practical importance.

Geoffrey Keynes, 1887-1982

30 The life of a medical student at a hospital can be pleasantly quiet if he chooses to be lazy, or tiringly exciting if he chooses otherwise.

Geoffrey Keynes, 1887-1982

31 Our immersion during residency has the most enduring influence on the way we practise surgery over the next 35 years.

Alexander J Walt, 1923-1996

32 You can not learn surgery sitting on your ass.

Ward Griffen

33 A teacher must not be the most facile surgeon, but he must be able to operate well, and he must remain an active clinician to command the respect of those whose education he shepherds.

Seymour I Schwartz

34   Nothing is more erroneous than the cliché: "those who can - do; those who can't - teach".

Seymour I Schwartz

35   If you take a son-of-a-bitch and educate him, you get an educated son-of-a-bitch.

Thomas Matthews Haizlip Sr

36   If the resident did it badly, make him re-do it; if he did it badly again, re-do it yourself.

37   Do not compromise the patient when operating from the left side - change sides if necessary.

38   Reprimand a resident who errs - fire the one who lies.

39   The only bad thing about being on call every other night is that you miss half of the educational opportunities.

40   For most medical students surgery is 70% scut work, 20% boredom, and 10% learning.

41   Medical student: "the only thing I learned during my surgery clerkship is that I am never going to have 'elective' surgery".

42   I was operating or resuscitating: the only two effective excuses for a missed conference.

43   Classical surgical education: see one, do one, teach one. Ideal surgical education: do one, do one, do one.

44   An expert surgeon: someone more than fifty miles from home with a carousel of slides.

45   50% of what you learn today will be obsolete in 5 years.

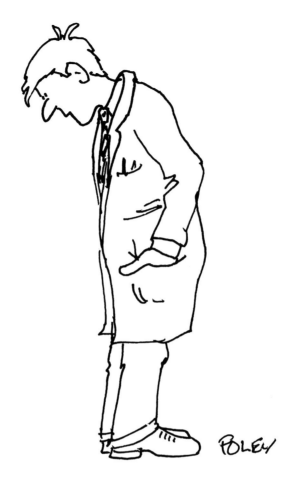

..... and also know something of the dangers and complications of the surgical undertaking.

From the editor

◆ A real surgeon shouts at his superiors - never at those below him.

Chapter 29

Empathy

1   Can you witness without distress the gasping for breath in an organic distress of the heart? If you can, you had better leave the profession: cast your diploma into the fire; you are not worthy to hold it.
Jacob M Da Costa, 1833-1900

2   As I esteem the honours, which have been conferred upon me, I regard that all worldly distinctions are as nothing in comparison with the hope that I may have been the means of reducing in some degree the sum of human misery.
Joseph Lister, 1827-1912

3   There is nothing we appreciate more than appreciation.
Marie von Ebner-Eschenbach, 1830-1916

4   A surgeon leaves his mark on the bodies of his patients, but they plow their marks in the furrows and wrinkles of his brow.
Rudolph Matas, 1860-1957

A surgeon leaves his mark on the bodies of his patients, but they plow their marks in the furrows and wrinkles of his brow.

Rudolph Matas, 1860-1957

5   On the sick bed we see man, as he is as well as who he is. He in turn, if we give wholly of ourselves, sees something of the secret in us. Here rather than in our societies, our laboratories, our hospitals, or our Universities, is our future. We'll keep it or lose it on the same field.

J Engelbert Dunphy, 1908-1981

6   Without a love of people, a doctor cannot function effectively for long and can never establish the requisite interpersonal relationships with patients ... a genuine affection for patients is essential if one is to absorb ingratitude without anger, weariness without irritability, criticism without rancor.

Alexander J Walt, 1923-1996

7   With a novelist, like a surgeon, you have to get a feeling that you've fallen into good hands - someone from whom you can accept the anesthetic with confidence.

Saul Bellow

Chapter 30

Errors

1   I have mistaken, but I have been mistaken less than other surgeons.
Guillaume Dupuytren, 1777-1835

2   I have made many mistakes myself ... the best surgeon, like the best general, is he who makes the fewest mistakes.
Astley Paston Cooper, 1768-1841

3   From the time of Hippocrates surgery has ever been the salvation of inner medicine. In inner medicine physicians have dwelt too much on dogmas, opinions and speculations; and too often their errors passed undiscovered to the grave. The surgeon, for his good, has had a sharper training; his errors hit him promptly in the face.
Thomas Clifford Allbutt, 1836-1925

4   What we call experience is often a dreadful list of ghastly mistakes.
J Chalmers Da Costa, 1863-1933

I have made many mistakes myself .... the best surgeon, like the best general, is he who makes the fewest mistakes.

Astley Paston Cooper, 1768-1841

5   More mistakes are made from want of a proper examination than for any other reason.

Russell John Howard, 1875-1942

6   A few observations and much reasoning leads to error; many observations and a little reasoning to truth.

Alexis Carrel, 1873-1944

7   The pilot is by circumstances allowed only one serious mistake, while the surgeon may commit many and not even recognize his own errors as such.

John S Lockwood, 1907-1950

8   To a patient after removing her breast (without a biopsy) for a benign lesion: "madam, I have made the most awful mistake, I've never before done such a thing in my whole life, I don't know how you can ever forgive me".

John Homans, 1877-1954

9   In the art of surgery, error is more likely to occur than in almost any other line of human endeavor.

Max Thorek, 1880-1960

10   While it is human to err, it is inhuman not to try, if possible, to protect those who entrust their lives into our hands from avoidable failures and danger.

Max Thorek, 1880-1960

11   The two unforgivable sins of surgery. The first great error in surgery is to operate unnecessarily; the second, to undertake an operation for which the surgeon is not sufficiently skilled technically.

Max Thorek, 1880-1960

12   You want a surgical team that faces each error, each mishap, straight up, names it, and takes steps to prevent its recurrence.

Francis D Moore, 1913-2001

13   Human error complicated by organisational factors is the main cause of accidents.

PO Nyström

14   It is usually the second mistake in response to the first mistake that does the patient in.

Clifton K Meador

15   In any given operation the source of error will never be determined if more than one person is involved.

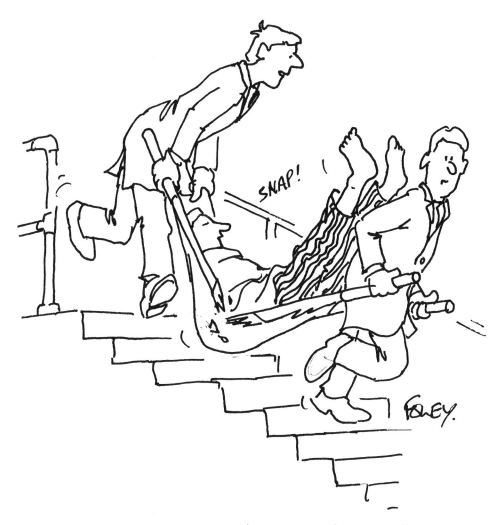

In any given operation the source of error will never be determined if more than one person is involved.

Physicians must particularly try to avoid being quacks. The fact that medicine is not an exact science favors quackery.

J Chalmers Da Costa, 1863-1933

Chapter 31

Ethics

1   And he should guard himself against drunkenness when he is to treat patients and ... if he has eaten onions or peas, or slept the previous night with an unclean woman, in the morning, against breathing into anyone's wound.
Heinrich von Pfolspeundt, ~1460

2   I say to all surgeons if there are two or several of them that they should never quarrel before the patient for that would frighten the patient very much.
Hieronymus Brunschwig, 1450-1512

3   You should not praise yourself but also not belittle the others. You should honour all men but particularly the priests and physicians so that you will have a good name.
Hieronymus Brunschwig, 1450-1512

4   He is continually operating in secret as a matter of necessity. The most sensible give the decision up to him; so that he is answerable to his own conscience, and to that alone.
Charles Bell, 1774-1842

5   I have noticed a tendency on the part of an occasional elderly and distinguished man to think that the rules of medical ethics were meant for young fellows just starting out, but not for him.

J Chalmers Da Costa, 1863-1933

6   Physicians must particularly try to avoid being quacks. The fact that medicine is not an exact science favors quackery.

J Chalmers Da Costa, 1863-1933

7   The tricks that are expected in a trade are disgraceful in a profession. The medical tradesman is being extremely low in the scale of animal creation, and he is responsible for most of the evils under which the profession labors.

J Chalmers Da Costa, 1863-1933

8   From the class of medical tradesmen come the prescribing and operating quack, the divider of fees, the recipient of commissions, the advertiser, the exploiter of formulas, the stealer of patients, the deceiver of sick persons, the swindler, the jealous vilifier of his professional brethren, the wholesale dealer in innuendo and calumny.

J Chalmers Da Costa, 1863-1933

9   The man who pays commission for cases has the effrontery of the confidence man, the skills of the pickpocket, the conscience of the burglar. It is a foul taint on the profession.

J Chalmers Da Costa, 1863-1933

10   He must avoid all advertising ... as well as issuing of private cards inviting the attention of persons affected with particular diseases ... avoid having on his letterheads ... the word "specialist" ... he must not promise to perform radical cures, must not publish cases of operations in the daily prints. He should not invite laypersons to be present at an operation; for it is a sort of method of advertising to do so.

J Chalmers Da Costa, 1863-1933

11   No physician may hold a patent for any surgical instrument or any medicine.

J Chalmers Da Costa, 1863-1933

12   What I object to ... is having "professional ethics" paraded like an innocent-eyed sacred cow, by men moved in their hearts by nothing more noble than good old-fashioned jealousy.

Max Thorek, 1880-1960

13   Medical ethics demand that we wait until we are consulted even when a case is screaming for treatment.

Ralph D Millard, Jr

14   Surgical Humanism as TPN ... the "T" stands for "tolerance" of our patients, especially at times of emotional stress; the "P" for "perspective" to enable us to see the much larger human picture framing the central pathology of the threatening lesion; and the "N" for "nurture" of our own talents so that we may have justifiable pride in the quality of our surgery and a fuller appreciation of our responsibilities to society.

Alexander J Walt, 1923-1996

15   In our concentration on spectacular cures, we have paid less attention to the concomitant burgeoning population of the deprived - the poor and our new large iatrogenic wave of medical immigrants, the aged. So we have a public greatly impressed by our technical achievements but disgruntled with what they regard as our careless, callous, thoughtless or even absent psychosocial sensitivities.

Alexander J Walt, 1923-1996

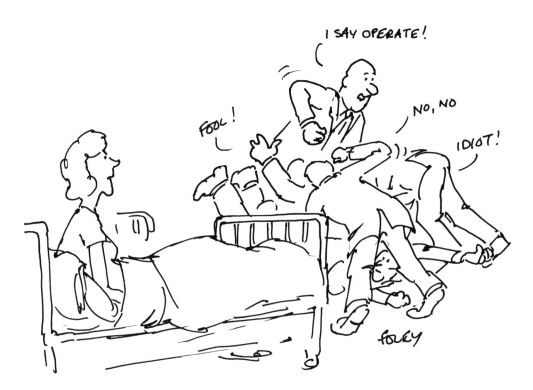

I say to all surgeons if there are two or several of them that they should never quarrel before the patient for that would frighten the patient very much.

Chapter 32

Experience

Good surgical judgment comes from experience and experience comes form poor surgical judgment.

1   The interns suffer not only from inexperience, but also from over experience.

William Stewart Halsted, 1852-1922

2   Each one of us, however old, is still an undergraduate in the school of experience. When a man thinks he has graduated he becomes a public menace.

J Chalmers Da Costa, 1863-1933

3   Age carries mental scars left by experience, which shortens vision, but age carries wisdom.

William J Mayo, 1861-1939

4   Experience is the great teacher; unfortunately, experience leaves mental scars, and scar tissue contracts.

William J Mayo, 1861-1939

5   From experience we should derive wisdom; but in surgery experience is never finished, and wisdom is never complete.

William Heneage Ogilvie, 1887-1971

6   A surgeon is a craftsman, basing his craft on a wide knowledge of human structure and biology, always gaining by experience of the results of his work.

Geoffrey Keynes, 1887-1982

7   Do not say "in my experience" until you have been in practice at least ten years.

Clifton K Meador

8   Good surgical judgment comes from experience and experience comes form poor surgical judgment.

Chapter 33

Feeding

God created man with a mouth, a stomach and gut - not a TPN line

Moshe Schein

1 In every disease it is a good sign when the patient's intellect is sound, and he is disposed to take whatever food is offered to him; but the contrary is bad.
Hippocrates, 460-377 BC

2 Some people never seem able to allow their patients to use the channels designed by nature to receive nourishment ... food and fluids given by the alimentary canal allow the tissues to select and keep what they want, and to reject what is harmful or surplus to requirements.
William Heneage Ogilvie, 1887-1971

3 In most conditions, foods that agree with the patients may be eaten, those which do not, should not be eaten.
Mark M Ravitch, 1910-1989

4 I tell my patients "I feed farts".
Frederick Foss

The patient may love you, but be sure that the spouse shares these feelings.

Chapter 34

Feelings

1 In truth, the anxiety of a surgeon, before an important operation, is the greatest any man can suffer ... and do not suppose that this belongs to a surgeon in his early practice only.

Charles Bell, 1774-1842

2 My calm feeling, that pleasant feeling of assurance and confidence that surgeons have when operations go well.

Francis D Moore, 1913-2001

3 The patient may love you, but be sure that the spouse shares these feelings.

From the editor

◆ After all, poetry and surgery are the same; usually based on gut-feeling rather than on objective data.

◆ When feeling guilty or insecure always blame the anesthetist, the patient or the resident.

Chapter 35

Future

1   The abdomen, the chest, and the brain will forever be shut from the intrusion of the wise and humane surgeon.

John Erichsen, 1818-1896

2   Manual skill has not appreciably improved in the last 50 years, and cannot improve much further. But manual skill is not the whole of surgery.

William Heneage Ogilvie, 1887-1971

3   What should we beg the boffins to produce for us? The first is a contrast medium excreted by the pancreas ... that will give a reasonably accurate estimate of pancreatic function, and allow the demonstration of obstruction to the ducts and of tumors at an early stage. The second is some systemic hemostatic that will arrest the bleeding from small vessels divided at operation.

William Heneage Ogilvie, 1887-1971

The day will certainly come when surgery will be done only to correct the effects of trauma and congenital abnormalities.

RH Meade

4   Surgery of the future will not tolerate the divorce of the hand from the brain and the surgery of the future will not be merely handicraft.

Isidor S Ravdin, 1894-1972

5   In the surgery of the future the individualist will be left by the roadside, for after all surgery is part of that broader field of experimental pathology to which all the medical sciences belong.

Isidor S Ravdin, 1894-1972

6   I sometimes see us moving through hospital corridors mournfully singing: "stitch that wound, open that tummy, do that 'trach', hurry up dummy, pass that 'scope', crack that head - hey, don't think - Halsted's dead."

Alexander J Walt, 1923-1996

7   Everything which can be done within the anatomical limits of the human body has been done. Nothing is left to be done, nothing is left to be dared. With great satisfaction we can sit back since we have reached the peak of surgery.

Jean-Louis Faire

8   As medicine has advanced, the role of surgery has decreased. The day will certainly come when surgery will be done only to correct the effects of trauma and congenital abnormalities.

RH Meade

9   **Phase 1** was the era of horror: cutting off, cutting open (butcher's trade). **Phase 2** was the era of extensive surgery. (I call it kilogram surgery.) **Phase 3** is the era of "tissue-sparing operations" (patient-friendly surgery), in which we are, I believe, right now ... another phase (**phase 4**) will follow where common surgery has ended. Possibly surgeons will then be responsible for trauma only. The surgeon will probably be referred to as a "tissue engineer" who manipulates cells and tissue instead of resecting organs, as suggested by Sir James Black, the Nobel Prize winner.

Hans Troidl

Chapter 36

General concepts

1 A physician well versed in the principles of surgery, and experienced in the practices of medicine, is alone capable of curing distempers, just as only a two-wheeled cart can be of service in a field of battle.

Sushruta, <8th century BC

2 Diseases which are not cured by medications are cured by iron; those which are not cured by iron are cured by fire; those which are not cured by fire are incurable.

Hippocrates, 460-377 BC

3 Extreme remedies are very appropriate for extreme diseases.

Hippocrates, 460-377 BC

4 It is wiser to attempt a doubtful remedy than to condemn the patient to certain death.

Celsus, 25BC-AD50

The operation is a silent confession to the surgeon's inadequacy.

John Hunter,

1728-1793

5   All the operations in surgery fall under two heads, separation and approximation. Approximation has to do with reduction and dressing of fractures ... of dislocations of joint ... of prolapsed intestine, uterus, or rectum, sutures of the abdomen ... division is concerned with simple incisions, circumcisions ... excisions of veins, amputation, scraping, smoothing, excisions with the saw.

Galen, 129-199AD

6   You know, my children, that surgical operations are divided into two classes: those that benefit the patient, and those that more often kill.

Albucasis, 936-1013

7   The surgeon who wishes to operate according to the rules should first frequent the places where able surgeons operate; follow with care their operations; fix them in his memory; and then practise by operating with these surgeons.

Henri de Mondeville, 1260-1320

8   Five things are proper to the duty of a chirurgeon: to take away that which is superfluous; to restore to their places such things as are displaced; to separate those things which are joined together; to join those that are separated; and to supply the defects of nature.

Ambroise Paré, 1510-1590

9   It is wiser to attempt a doubtful remedy, than absolutely to despair.

Lorenz Heister, 1683-1758

10   The operation is a silent confession to the surgeon's inadequacy.

John Hunter, 1728-1793

11   The surgeon is dealing with the most divine of all professions: to heal without wonders, and to perform wonders without words.

Johann Wolfgang von Goethe, 1749-1832

12   The pleasure of a physician is little, the gratitude of patients is rare, and even rarer is material reward, but these things will never deter the student who feels the call within him.

Theodor Billroth, 1829-1894

13   In surgery, eyes first and most; fingers next and little; tongue last and least.

Humphrey George Murray, 1820-1896

14   The most important result of any surgical operation is a live patient.

Charles H Mayo, 1865-1939

15   Surgery may not require brains or bring a fortune, but it is the best job in the world.

William Heneage Ogilvie, 1887-1971

16   Always do the things you are afraid to do - next time it will be much easier.

Charles FM Saint, 1886-1973

17   A good operation depends on conservatism, consistent with efficiency; simplicity of technique; operative skill, which includes gentleness, dexterity, and careful speed; and maximal benefit from minimal interference.

Charles FM Saint, 1886-1973

18   For the difficult surgery of today, a sturdy pair of legs is also an indispensable necessity!

Owen H Wangensteen, 1898-1981

19   Surgery, like war, is hard ... but it is better than war. It saves lives and binds men and women of good will together in deepest friendship.

J Engelbert Dunphy, 1908-1981

20   The surgeon must operate by sight, not by faith.

Rodney Maingot, 1893-1982

21   When there is multiplicity of operations for one condition, it proves that either none is effective, or all are effective.

Mark M Ravitch, 1910-1989

22   In massive insults to the organism, treat the patient for the insult, without waiting for the response to the insult.

Mark M Ravitch, 1910-1989

23 An operation is an assault on a fellow human being - legalised, but nonetheless an assault. In a sense, today the license to kill is given by society only to surgeons.

Alexander J Walt, 1923-1996

24 The most important thing before an operation is what I think about it the night before.

Francis D Moore, 1913-2001

25 All that is wrong cannot be righted - be sure the wrongs are rightly sighted.

Francis D Moore, 1913-2001

26 Surgery does the ideal thing - it separates the patient from his disease. It puts the patient back to bed and the disease in a bottle.

Logan Clendening

27 Moral of the story: a tincture of time is a wonderful medicine; operate on the patient, not on the x-ray; the messier the case the longer the ileus; many patients will need a "trial by fire" during a complicated course - if they fail they go to the OR; always try to avoid operating on lawyers.

George Portilla

28 People believing in the "immaculate conception" will believe in everything!

Friedrich C Lang

29 To a lot of surgeons, surgery is, after all, like masturbation.

Rui Sequeira

30 Everything in surgery is complicated until one learns to do it well, then it is easy.

Robert E Condon

31 But after all, when all is said and done, the king of all topics is the operation.

Irvin S Cobb

32   The track record of most surgical procedures for disorders having a physiological abnormality but with exaggerated psychiatric overtones is a dismal one of failed surgical endeavour.

MRB Keighley

33   The joy of surgery: 1. The pleasure of helping a sick person get better; 2. The discovery of new knowledge; 3. The pleasure of teaching; 4. The creative use of the hands.

Frank C Spencer

34   Winning is over emphasised. The only time it is really important is in surgery and war.

Al McGuire

35   Life as surgery, is like a dog sled. If you ain't top dog the view does not change.

36   A minor operation is what the other person has.

37   Surgery is to be done, not to have.

38   An operative list is like a chess game series: you have to play one case at a time without regard to the results of the previous case or for the difficulty of the one to follow.

From the editor

◆ The larger the operation, the greater is the trauma. The greater is the trauma, the stronger is the SIRS. The stronger is the SIRS, the sicker is the patient; the sicker is the patient, the higher is his M & M.

Giants walked

these floors -

always two years

before you arrived.

Chapter 37

Giants & Greatness

1   The moderns are, in relation to the ancients, as a dwarf placed on the shoulders of a giant; he sees all that the giant perceives plus a little more.

Henri de Mondeville, 1260-1320

2   Lister saw the vast importance of the discoveries of Pasteur. He saw it because he was watching on the heights, and he was watching there alone.

Thomas Clifford Allbutt, 1836-1925

3   On the roll call which, in letters of gold, bears the names of the saviors of mankind, no man is more worthy of remembrance than Lister.

Berkeley Moynihan, 1865-1936

4   As I look back on these men who influenced me so greatly, I realize that their influence lay not in their craftsmanship, but in their high qualities of mind.

William J Mayo, 1861-1939

5   About Rudolf Nissen: "somehow he reminds me of a surgical Paganini".

Max Thorek, 1880-1960

6   All surgical roads lead to John Hunter. In the search of those first principles which have guided great men their successors should probe the working of their mind rather than their technical successes.

James Learmonth, 1895-1967

7   On John Hunter: "the fire of his genius threw a beam into the darkness ahead and lit the torch of inquiry that has been the glory of British surgery".

William Heneage Ogilvie, 1887-1971

8   In judging a surgeon we must consider qualities of the head, the heart, and the hand. Greatness of hand is greatness of the hour, lasting only while the skills last and forgotten within a few months of death and retirement. Greatness of the head leads to a secure place during life and an honoured memory afterwards. Greatness of the heart brings a personal influence on patients and pupils and a name that will live among them for one or more generations. When greatness of head and heart combine together they bring immortality.

William Heneage Ogilvie, 1887-1971

9   If the ability ... to leave a living memory rather than a bibliography is the test of greatness, then personality is the most important attribute of a great surgeon.

William Heneage Ogilvie, 1887-1971

10   What, then, are the marks of the really great surgeon? He must, I think, be judged on at least five separate counts ... my principle is to award marks on each count: 10 for knowledge, 30 for original work, 30 for clinical judgment, 20 for operating, and 10 for teaching and writing. To reach the first class a surgeon must obtain 80.

William Heneage Ogilvie, 1887-1971

11 Most eminent men are in a large degree self-made and have pursued their subject from the attraction before them, not from stimulus behind. You cannot create this talent. You may indeed give it opportunity but you cannot force it.

Edward D Churchill, 1895-1972

12 As Moynihan's assistant I felt as a young sculptor might have felt finding himself unexpectedly apprenticed to Michelangelo.

Geoffrey Keynes, 1887-1982

13 On Alfred Blalock (1899-1964): "with the passage of time, his shadow continues to lengthen and a day seldom passes but my thoughts return to him, usually with a single question 'how would he manage this?'"

David Sabiston

14 The giants of today may be a little different from prior giants. But not in the essentials ... a giant is a giant because he is wiser, more imaginative, more tenacious, more industrious and more effective than these around him. Furthermore, he will always be recognized as a giant, even in a society in which we are all considered equal.

M Mark Veto

15 On William Halsted: "ashes rest in Brooklyn; the flame burns on".

Seymour I Schwartz

16 Giants walked these floors - always two years before you arrived.

Chapter 38

No guts no glory.

Glory & Fame

1   The glory of surgeons is like that of actors, which lasts only for their own lifetime and can no longer be appreciated once they have passed away. Actors and surgeons ... are all heroes of the moment.
Honore de Balzac, 1799-1850

2   Medical fame, after all, and at its best, is limited to a very restricted audience. Libraries are crowded with the biographies of soldiers, statesmen, monarchs, orators, scientists, inventors, navigators, explorers, bank burglars, detectives, and philanthropists; and if a library happens to contain a book or two upon physicians, these books will be found tossed unread on the topmost shelf.
J Chalmers Da Costa, 1863-1933

3   The glory of medicine is that it is constantly moving forward, that there is always more to learn.
William J Mayo, 1861-1939

The surgeon must have the heart of a lion, the eyes of a hawk, and the hands of a woman.

John Halle,

1529-1568

Chapter 39

Hands & Manual Skills

1   The nails shoud be neither longer nor shorter than the points of the fingers; and the surgeon should practise with the extremities of the fingers, the index-finger being usually turned to the thumb.

Hippocrates, 460-377 BC

2   Now a surgeon should be youthful or at any rate nearer youth than age; with a strong and steady hand which never trembles and ready to use the left hand as well as the right.

Celsus, 25BC-AD50

3   In the part of medicine that cures by hand, it is obvious that all improvement comes chiefly from this, even if assisted somewhat in other ways.

Celsus, 25BC-AD50

4   He who works with his hands is a labourer. He who works with his head and his hands is a craftsman.

St. Francis of Assisi, 1181-1226

5   He should have well-formed limbs, especially the hands, the fingers long and slender, agile and not trembling; all the other limbs strong, in order to be able to execute in manly fashion.

Henri de Mondeville, 1260-1320

6   The surgeon must have the heart of a lion, the eyes of a hawk, and the hands of a woman.

John Halle, 1529-1568

7   But the quality which is considered of the highest order in surgical operations is self-possession; the head must always direct the hand.

Astley Paston Cooper, 1768-1841

8   The surgeon must have no poison on his hands.

Ignaz Semmelweis, 1818-1865

9   A good surgeon operates with his hand, not with his heart.

Alexandre Dumas Pére, 1802-1870

10   To intrude an unskilled hand into such a piece of devine mechanism as the human body is indeed a fearful responsibility.

Joseph Lister, 1827-1912

11   I would like to see the day when somebody would be appointed surgeon somewhere who had no hands, for the operative part is the least part of the work.

Harvey Williams Cushing, 1869-1939

12   The finger is superior to all instruments. Covered with parts soft and supple, it causes little pain, it can be placed in narrow spaces; flexible, it conforms to various parts; sensitive, it permits the appreciation of the variations in resistance of the parts percussed.

Henri A Hartmann, 1860-1952

13   Even in plastic surgery, where meticulous artistry might be thought to be the first consideration, the best results are obtained by those who think, plan, and prepare, rather than by those who perform with the self-conscious skill of the trapeze artist.

William Heneage Ogilvie, 1887-1971

14   Many of the greatest surgeons were but indifferent operators; and conversely many, perhaps most, brilliant technicians have been second-rate surgeons, earning the meretricious applause of the virtuoso while their artistry was at its heyday - forgotten like the discarded prima donna as soon as their skill passed its zenith.

William Heneage Ogilvie, 1887-1971

15   The dexterous hand must not be allowed to reach before imperfect judgment.

Zachary Cope, 1881-1974

16   Don't put your hands before your mind.

Nick Mendel

17   Busy hands are happy.

Jerry McCold

18   He is ambidextrous - equally clumsy with both hands.

Gail Waldby

19   Surgeons behave like Poncius Pilatos: they wash their hands before acting.

Chapter 40

Heart

1 It is impossible to save a patient when ... the heart ... has been pierced. When the heart is penetrated, much blood issues, the pulse fades away, the colour is extremely pallid, cold and malodorous sweats burst out as if the body had been wetted by dew, the extremities become cold and death quickly follows.

Celsus, 25BC-AD50

2 When a perforation penetrated in one of the cardiac ventricles, they died on the spot, mainly by blood loss, and even faster if the left ventricle was injured. When the penetrating object did not pass through the cardiac cavity but stopped at the cardiac muscle, some of the wounded gladiators lived through the very day...as well the following night; they eventually died later because of an inflammation of the heart.

Galen, 129-199AD

Anyone who would attempt to operate on the heart should lose the respect of his colleagues.

Theodor Billroth, 1829-1894

3   The heart is the chief mansion of the soul, the organ of vital capacity, the beginning of life, the foundation of the vital spirits ... the first to live the last to die.

Ambroise Paré, 1510-1590

4   Often times an abundance of moisture therein (the pericardium), which causes suffocation and overwhelms the heart.

Jean Riolan, 1580-1657

5   A few years ago it was considered as a fact placed beyond any doubt that wounds of the heart were necessarily mortal ... even at present, in spite of the number of facts and observations collected at the Hotel Dieu ... the contrary opinion is far from being generally admitted.

Guillaume Dupuytren, 1777-1835

6   To hear a murmur is a very different matter from feeling the blood itself pouring back over one's finger.

Henry Sessions Souttar, ~1875

7   Anyone who would attempt to operate on the heart should lose the respect of his colleagues.

Theodor Billroth, 1829-1894

8   First repair of cardiac wound: "it was very disquieting to see the heart pause in diastole with each pass of the needle ... the heart gave a laboured beat, and then resumed with forceful contractions as we breathed a sigh of relief".

Ludwig Rehn, ~1896

9   Let me speak once more my conviction that by means of the cardiorrhapy, many lives can be saved that were previously counted as lost.

Ludwig Rehn, ~1896

10   Surgery of the heart has probably reached the limits set by nature to all surgery: no new method and no new discovery can overcome the natural difficulties that attend a wound of the heart.

James Paget, 1814-1899

11   The suggestion to suture a wound to the heart, although made in all seriousness, scarcely deserves mention.

F Riedinger, 1845-1918

12   Any operation which reduces the mortality of a given injury from 90 to about 63 per cent is entitled to a permanent place in surgery, and ... every wound of the heart should be operated upon immediately.

Luther Leonidas Hill Jr

Nine of every ten

men have piles.

Chapter 41

Hemorrhoids

1 It is not clear if these haemorrhoids are of the variety which should be excised or not, since there are people in whom they have once been surgically extirpated and in whom other haemorrhoids develop.
Moses Maimonides, 1135-1204

2 Kiss your haemorrhoids goodbye.
David Dunn

3 Hemorrhoids are an epiphenomenon.
Antonio Longo

4 Nine of every ten men have piles.

5 After (open) haemorrhoidectomy if wound shape is clover then the problem is over - if dahlia, then it is a problem.

Chapter 42

Hernia

1   The testicle having been thus cleared is to be gently returned through the incision along with the veins and arteries and its cord; and it must be seen that blood does not drop down into the scrotum, or a clot remain anywhere.

Celsus, 25BC-AD50

2   When a rupture occurs in the groin, and part of the intestine and omentum comes down into the scrotum ... let him lie on his back ... and ... hold his breath till the intestine ... comes out; then put it back with your finger. Then below the hernia over the pubic bone, mark a semicircle ... then heat a cautery ... when it is white hot and emits sparks ... have the assistant put his hand over the place to prevent the exit of the intestine ... then apply the cautery to the mark ... and hold it until it reaches the bone ... if you do not bring the cauterisation down to the bone your operation will not be successful ... the patient should lie on his back for forty days so that the wound may cicatrise.

Albucasis, 936-1013

You can judge the worth of a surgeon by the way he does a hernia.

Thomas Fairbank,

1876-1961

3   Permit the testicle to redescend to its place, and do not dream in any fashion of extirpating it, as do some stupid and ignorant doctors who know nothing; but take the spermatic cord itself and the conduit through which the intestine descends to the place which the testicle occupies ... and tie completely this conduit and the spermatic cord ...

William of Salicet, 1210-1277

4   No disease of the human body, belonging to the province of the surgeon, requires in its treatment a better combination of accurate anatomical knowledge, with surgical skill, than a hernia in all its variety.

Astley Paston Cooper, 1768-1841

5   Always explore in cases of persistent vomiting if a lump, however small, is found occupying one of the abdominal rings and its nature is uncertain.

Augustus Charles Bernays, 1854-1907

6   In order to achieve a radical cure (of inguinal hernia) it is absolutely essential to restore those conditions in the area of the hernial orifice, which exist under normal conditions.

Edoardo Bassini, 1844-1924

7   You can judge the worth of a surgeon by the way he does a hernia.

Thomas Fairbank, 1876-1961

8   There is no doubt that the first appearance of the mammal, with his unexplained need to push his testicles out of their proper home into the air, made a mess of the three layered abdominal wall that had done the reptiles well for 200 million years.

William Heneage Ogilvie, 1887-1971

9   Numbness is better than neuropathy.

Francis C Usher 1908-1980

10   The history of hernia is the history of surgery.

Lloyd Nyhus & Robert E Condon

11   For the understanding of the etiology, the pathology, the clinical manifestations and, particularly, the surgical repair of an indirect inguinal hernia, a profound knowledge of the anatomy of this region is indispensable.

Frank Netter

12   Dr. Erle Peacock (~1926) ruled: "a hernia is an abnormal protrusion of an organ through an opening!" Whereupon the intern stuck out his tongue at Dr. Peacock saying, "so would this be a hernia, sir?".

Peter Bradshaw

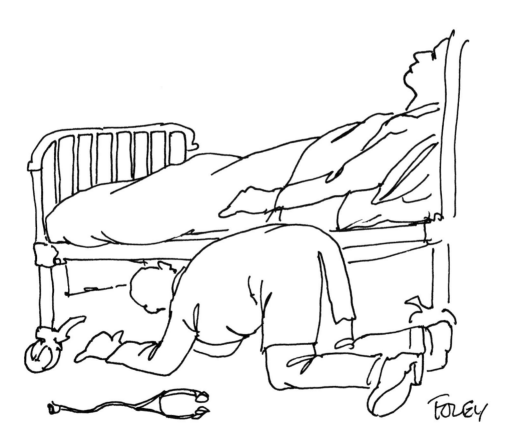

..... the first appearance of the mammal, with his unexplained need to push his testicles out of their proper home into the air.....

There are only

two periods in the

history of surgery

- before Lister and

after Lister.

Harvey Graham,

~ 1939

Chapter 43

History

1 It has been said that there are only two periods in the history of surgery - before Lister and after Lister.

Harvey Graham, ~1939

2 In the study of some apparently new problems we often make progress by reading the work of the great men of the past.

Charles H Mayo, 1865-1939

3 The most precious heritage of our profession lies in the noble traditions. What has been accomplished does not die, but too often, alas, the personality of those who have handed the torch from one generation to another soon fades into oblivion.

Harvey Williams Cushing, 1869-1939

4   For the records show, to one who reads with honesty, how old is our newest knowledge, how painfully and proudly we struggle to discoveries, which, instead of being new truth, are only rediscoveries of lost knowledge.

Max Thorek, 1880-1960

5   In reality there is no way to separate today's surgery and our practice from the experiences of all the surgeons who have preceded us.

Ira M Rutkow

6   It is a magnificent adventure for the budding surgeon to recognize what he or she is currently learning within the context of past and present social, cultural, and economic institutions.

Ira M Rutkow

No incision

signifies

indecision,

provided you can

decide.

Moshe Schein

Chapter 44

Incisions

1 Where the surgery is performed by a single incision, you must make it a quick one; for since the person being cut usually suffers pain, this suffering should last for the least time possible .... When many incisions are necessary, you must employ a slow surgery, for a surgeon that was fast would make the pain sustained and great, whereas intervals provide a break for the patients.
Hippocrates, 460-377 BC

2 Surgeons must be very careful when they take the knife. Underneath their fine incisions stirs the culprit - LIFE!
Emily Dickinson, 1830-1886

3 The incision must be as long as necessary and as short as possible.
Theodor Kocher, 1841-1917

4 Pray before surgery, but remember God will not alter a faulty incision.
Arthur H Keeney, ~1920

5   Students come to think that all a surgeon needs to know is how to adorn himself in robes and boots, how to cleanse his hands by some process of extraordinary severity and complexity, and how to make an exploratory incision.

J Chalmers Da Costa, 1863-1933

6   Cut with the scalpel, don't scratch.

Mark M Ravitch, 1910-1989

7   Wounds heal across, not in length, but the longer the wound the greater the tension required to close it.

Mark M Ravitch, 1910-1989

8   A senior surgeon, when called to a difficult operation, first enlarges the incision, second - he begins to think.

Denis M Arkhipov

9   It is better if the patient goes to the plastic surgeon after an operation, with a large scar, than to the pathologist with a small one.

Denis M Arkhipov

10   Incisions heal from side to side, not end to end, but length does matter.

11   Big surgeon - big incision.

12   Little incisions are for surgeons with little brains.

13   The incision should not look like charcoal - use the diathermy sparingly.

14   When entering the abdomen, your finger is the best and safest instrument.

15   Two good incisions are better than one poorly placed.

The lesser the indication, the greater the complication.

Chapter 45

Indications

1   The most important decisions in surgery concern operations, whether they shall be done, when they shall be done, and what form they should take. In most operations there is only one best time, and often that best time is reached or passed before a diagnosis can be made...
   William Heneage Ogilvie, 1887-1971

2   The feasibility of an operation is not the best indication for its performance.
   Henry Cohen, 1900-1977

3   The decision for operation cannot be made by plebiscite.
   Mark M Ravitch, 1910-1989

4   The basic guideline is "would you have this done to yourself, your wife, your child, your parent?"
   Mark M Ravitch, 1910-1989

5   The lesser the indication, the greater the complication.

Chapter 46

Infection

1   The wound should be treated in such a way as to produce suppuration as quickly as possible.
    Hippocrates, 460-377 BC

2   It is not necessary ... as all modern surgeons profess, that pus should be generated in wounds. No error can be greater than this.
    Hugh of Lucca, 1160-1257

3   Many more surgeons know how to cause suppuration than to heal a wound.
    Henri de Mondeville, 1260-1320

4   He should bind with white cloths, for if they are not clean, harm results. He should also wash his hands before he treats anyone.
    Heinrich von Pfolspeundt, ~1460

5   Inflammation is not itself considered a disease but a salutary operation ... but when it cannot accomplish that salutary purpose ... it does mischief.
    John Hunter, 1728-1793

Every operation in surgery is an experiment in bacteriology.

Berkeley Moynihan, 1865-1936

6   The fear of "hospitalism" is past and the surgical patient no longer is exposed to more chances of death than the English soldier on the field of Waterloo.

James Y Simpson, 1811-1870

7   The time will assuredly arrive when peritonitis will not kill, because we will learn that the effusions in the peritoneal cavity may be as safely evacuated as those in the pleural cavity.

James Marion Sims, 1813-1883

8   Little if any face is placed by any enlightened or experienced surgeon on this side of the Atlantic in the so-called carbolic acid treatment of Professor Lister.

Samuel Gross, 1805-1884

9   Had I had the honour of being a surgeon, impressed as I am with the dangers of exposure to germs and microbes scattered on the surface of all objects, particularly in hospitals, not only would I use perfectly clean instruments, but after washing my hands with the greatest care and submitting them to a rapid flaming, which would cause no more discomfort than a smoker feels in passing a burning coal from one hand to another, I would use charpie, bandages, sponges previously exposed to air at 130° to 150°C temperature.

Louis Pasteur, 1822-1895

10   The only solution for endemic infection was complete demolition, repeated in regular intervals of every hospital afflicted with hospitalism.

John Erichsen, 1818-1896

11   When thou findest a purulent swelling with the apex elevated, sharply defined and of a round form, then sayest thou, "it is a purulent tumour which is growing in the flesh. I must treat the disease with a knife".

George Ebers, 1837-1898, surgical papyrus

12   The real danger in fever is not the pyrexia but the poison causing it.

Augustus Charles Bernays, 1854-1907

13   Fever is, in a measure, a beneficial process operating to protect the economy.

Augustus Charles Bernays, 1854-1907

14   View with anxiety any case of sepsis, which has a low temperature.
Augustus Charles Bernays, 1854-1907

15   My house surgeon ... acting under my instructions ... laid a piece of lint dipped in liquid carbolic acid upon the wound, and applied ... splints ... the remarkable retardation of suppuration, and the immediate conversion of the compound fracture into a simple fracture with a superficial sore, were more encouraging facts.
Joseph Lister, 1827-1912

16   In using the expression "dressed antiseptically" I do not mean merely "dressed with an antiseptic" but "dressed so as to ensure absence of putrefaction".
Joseph Lister, 1827-1912

17   I do not expect my contemporaries to accept all my doctrines, but I look to the coming generation to adopt and perfect them.
Joseph Lister, 1827-1912

18   Every operation in surgery is an experiment in bacteriology.
Berkeley Moynihan, 1865-1936

19   Many cocci, particularly pneumococci and the cocci found in pyaemia, are stained intensely, whilst some few other bacteria, such as typhoid, are decolorized.
Christian Gram, 1853-1938

20   The phagocyte is the best antiseptic.
Alexander Fleming, 1881-1955

21   As long as surgical infections exist, surgeons must make never-ending efforts to control them. It may be described as a time when science and art can absolutely prevent bacteria from gaining a foothold in the human body and can abruptly terminate their activity, if they have already become established.
Frank L Meleney, 1889-1963

22   Drain pus through the shortest route.
Mark M Ravitch, 1910-1989

23   To isolate patients is to invite neglect.

Mark M Ravitch,1910-1989

24   These bacteria are called *Escherichia coli* in honour of Theodor Escherich, a scientist of the nineteenth century.

Francis D Moore, 1913-2001

25   The mechanical control of the source of infection, while itself nonbiologic, determines the extent of the host biologic response to the disease.

Ronald V Maier

26   Sepsis is not an antibiotic-deficiency syndrome.

John Marshall

27   In peritonitis - source control is above all.

28   Why it's fun to drain abscesses? Because you can't infect pus.

29   Infected devices? When in doubt, take it out.

From the editor

◆ The most novel antibiotics and the best supportive care are meaningless, if principles of source control are not adhered to with obsessiveness.

◆ "Signs of pus somewhere, signs of pus nowhere else, signs of pus there - under the diaphragm". This was 100% true when I was a student, 50% true when I was a resident. Today it is irrelevant. And Mark M Ravitch added: "...and masked by antibiotics".

◆ Infectious disease specialists: don't they know that an abscess reflects the victory of the peritoneal defences?

◆ If you sample/culture shit, you get shitty results which fill your brain with shit and then you bother us with absolute shit during this snowy weekend, when we want to see white snow and not brown shit.

◆ People claim that lavage is the solution to pollution by dilution of the contaminants, but remember that macrophages do not swim well.

◆ Attempting trans-laparoscopic management of complicated post-operative peritonitis is like making love to a fully dressed harem woman.

Chapter 47

Innovations & Gimmicks

Fingers replace brains, and handicraft outruns science.

Edward W Archibald, 1872-1945

New "surgical innovation" as a revolution

Surgeons as all human beings express a few limited patterns of attitude. One could compare a surgical innovation to a political revolution (e.g. the French, the October in Russia or that of the National-Socialists in Germany during the 1930s). To simplify matters let me identify six main patterns of attitude. The revolution in our case will be the "anal stapling procedure" (ASP) also known as PPH (procedure for prolapsed hemorrhoids).

The true revolutionists

Those are the few true innovators; they developed the new method; they introduced it. If it wins, their fame and wealth is secure; if they lose, then they are back to obscurity. Thus, they are ready even to die for an idea, which may shine a new light on the anus for a thousand years.

The true intellectuals

Those are the very few who join the revolution only after assessing its value from inside out. They are ready to join it, but once they see that its direction is false, they would quit, ready to pay for the consequences. Those are the surgeons who would go and learn ASP from the true revolutionists and then submit the innovation to the scientific scrutiny of level I studies always ready to abort and confess that the revolution was wrong. This is clearly a tiny minority. By the way those are also the people who use the term anal cushions instead of hemorrhoids.

The profiteers

Those are the sort of people who would join any revolution as long as they can have a personal gain, be it a better position, academic advantage, power, money and prestige. They would join any revolution irrespective of its nature. They will use the ASP, correctly or incorrectly, on anyone who has an anus in order to gain more patients, more money and simply to have fun. They do not represent a minority.

The reactionaries

They tend to oppose and resist any revolution. They are happy with the old order whatever it is. They do not want to learn anything new. They were doing conventional pile surgery; their patients are happy, right? So why change? No, they are not active counter-revolutionaries but simply, they do not care and are passive. They are not members of the resistance, nor are they collaborators. They make a significant portion of the surgical community.

The counter-revolutionists.

Those are the surgeons who perceive from the beginning that the revolution is false or wrong. They fight against it. Those are the ones who die on the guillotine, in the "gulags" or in the "camps". Occasionally they are wrong but usually they fight for the right cause sensing that the new procedure is dangerous, and gimmicky, and has to be aborted.

The masses

This is the vast majority. They would sit tight on the fence, waiting to see how things develop and who will win. They care about bringing bread to their families and cure to their patients. They would support the revolution only after they see it has succeeded. Unfortunately, they may join it at some stage even if they know it is wrong and evil. They are forced to do so; they do not want to die together with the counter-revolutionists for they are not heroes. "If everybody does ASP I have to do it as well".

Being humans, surgeons' attitudes to surgical innovations follows certain fixed patterns. Are we not predictable? To which group do you belong?

1   That which is new at this time will one day be ancient; as what is ancient was once new. It is not the length of time which gives value to things, it is their own excellency.

Augustine Belloste, 1645-1730

2   If you are too fond of new remedies, first you will not cure your patients; secondly, you will have no patients to cure.

Astley Paston Cooper, 1768-1841

3   Every idea is an incitement ... eloquence may set fire to reason.

Oliver Wendell Holmes, 1809-1894

4   There must be a final limit to the development of manipulative surgery. The knife cannot always have fresh fields for conquest; and although methods of practice may be modified and varied, and even improved to some extent, it must be within a certain limit.

John Erichsen, 1818-1896

5   The seeming exactness of a mechanical device appeals much more strongly to certain minds than a process of reasoning.

James Mackenzie, 1853-1925

6   There are fashions in surgery just as there are in morals, millinery, religion, and war boats. They are just as transitory and often just as bizarre.

J Chalmers Da Costa, 1863-1933

7   Fingers replace brains, and handicraft outruns science.

Edward W Archibald, 1872-1945

8   The introduction of an instrument is more or less of an evil, never to be resorted to, unless a greater evil be present, which its employment may probably remedy.

Harold Thompson, 1897-?

9   As he picks up his beautiful new tool, however, it is well for the modern biologist to remind himself how subtly and completely a fascination for gadgets can betray sound sense.

William T Salter, 1901-1952

10   We must also keep in mind that discoveries are usually not made by one man alone, but that many brains and many hands are needed before discovery is made for which one man receives the credit.

Henry E Sigerist, 1891-1957

11   The great publicity, which certain operative procedures receive ... is to be blamed for a good many of the unfortunate results which follow injudicious surgery. They are often demanded in the belief that they are an advance, and the local surgeon is tempted to comply with such demands ... and to perform an operation which is unfamiliar to him - very frequently and with unfortunate results.

Max Thorek, 1880-1960

12   It usually requires a considerable time to determine with certainty the virtues of a new method of treatment and usually still longer to ascertain the harmful effects.

Alfred Blalock, 1899-1964

13   Surgeons are enthusiasts or they would not be surgeons. They tend to overvalue each new procedure propounded to them, and to extend its field of application beyond that intended by its author, often to use it in cases in which it is unsuitable. The man who sounds a note of caution is branded as a Jeremiah, a spoil-sport, a back number; yet in the end his views are usually shown to have been right.

William Heneage Ogilvie, 1887-1971

14   Medicine consists of science, wisdom, and technology. We teach the science; we ignore the study of human behavior from which wisdom could derive; and we profess to despise technology though we see it all around us.

Robert Platt, 1900-1978

15   I found myself again showing signs of suffering from Lord Taylor's "salmon syndrome": swimming against the stream.

Geoffrey Keynes, 1887-1982

16   In general, if a technique has been adequately reported in a major journal, but was then not persistently followed up by its creators with a succession of papers confirming the original success, and was not picked up by others, the conclusion may safely be drawn that the procedure was defective or unattractive, and had probably been tried by others, who found it wanting, perhaps without bothering even to publish. There are exceptions to this.

Mark M Ravitch, 1910-1989

17   We have at times too long from custom persisted in procedures no longer justified. We have sometimes not examined closely enough new procedures that have ultimately proved useful.

Mark M Ravitch, 1910-1989

18   New equipment and new procedures may improve medical care, but seldom decrease cost.

Mark M Ravitch, 1910-1989

19   New ideas seldom have the simplicity of a switched on light bulb.

Thomas Starzl

20   We, the surgeons, are the most gimmick-conscious group of suckers of any other professionals in the world.

Eric Frykberg

21   We seem to have replaced cheap & effective with expensive & mediocre.

Anil Thakur

22   An increasing worship of instrument for its own sake sometimes leads to enslavement by it.

David Seegal

23   We do not need a compass to find our way home.

24   A fool with a tool is still a fool.

25   After some of those advanced minimally invasive procedures the patient advances to the recovery room but the surgeon may need an ICU.

From the editor

◆   We in the USA have become an excessively invasive surgical society. Too many Swan-Ganzs, too many coronary angioplasties for MI, and too many PEGS/gastrostomies. The late NY cardiologist Bernard Lown wrote: "the reason for this shift includes a romance with mindless technology, which is embraced largely to maximize income. Since it is unnecessary to spend much time with patients ... it opens floodgates for endless procedures".

◆   Unfortunately, medicine becomes more and more invasive; lives are saved, lives are being lost; the net results remain the same, but at a much higher price.

Chapter 48

International surgery

1   There are many learned men in Germany who could further medical knowledge but they are so taken up with their useless labours and with poring over old books that they cannot be made to know that the real basis of medicine is "love thy neighbour".
Paracelsus, 1493-1541

2   What I inveigh against is a cursed spirit of intolerance, conceived in distrust and bred in ignorance, that makes the mental attitude perennially antagonistic, even bitterly antagonistic to everything foreign, that subordinates everywhere the race to nation, forgetting the higher claims of human brotherhood.
William Osler, 1849-1919

3   Americans, newly arrived in Austria, we were greatly amused at seeing perhaps a dozen clamps left hanging in a wound of the neck while the operator proceeded with his dissection, and were inclined to

International congresses. There flowery speakers of all nations convene and infect one another.

August Bier,

1861-1949

ridicule the method as being untidy and uncouth. Slowly it dawned on us that we in America were novices in the art as well as the science of surgery.

William Stewart Halsted, 1852-1922

4 There is a fashion in the way we do things surgically as truly as there is a fashion in neckties and bonnets. The world has adopted the custom of taking the fashions of its clothing from Paris; and the medical world has largely adopted the custom of taking the fashion from Germany. In determining if a German fashion is true it is a good rule to let it pass through England and see what the common sense British mind has to say of it and then weigh up the two views.

J Chalmers Da Costa, 1863-1933

5 The problem before us is so to exchange information, and so to educate men through travel that there shall develop a final, cosmopolitan system of medicine which will combine the best elements to be found in all countries.

Charles H Mayo, 1865-1939

6 Since the object of travel is primarily self-improvement, time should not be wasted looking for things done badly and for things to criticize.

William J Mayo, 1861-1939

7 International congresses. There flowery speakers of all nations convene and infect one another.

August Bier, 1861-1949

8 It is worth it to go half-way round the world to watch another surgeon at work, and to bring home the requisite tools for the job.

Thomas Dunhill, 1876-1957

9 American hospital? With all these strange faces and these foreign accents? A thousand times yes … For here, safe from the madness which engulfs the world, meet some of the great minds of European clinics, sharing … knowledge and their experience in a fellowship which is the very essence of democracy.

Max Thorek, 1880-1960

10   National surgery is modified by national temperament ... German surgeons bring to their opportunities a thoroughness and industry that are wholly admirable ... French surgeons lose by a certain intolerance and contempt for the knowledge and culture of other nations, whose advances they rarely assimilate ... the British surgeon ... if he seeks public recognition ... knows that he is more likely to obtain it by a beautiful motor car or a socially-minded wife, than by originality or skill.

William Heneage Ogilvie, 1887-1971

11   It is characteristic of continental surgery that professional and national recognition is synonymous. The great surgeon is, at the same time, an honoured servant of the State and a familiar figure to the people. There is no counterpart to two types that are met in England; on the one hand the idol of the public, whose name is a household word and whose portrait is news, but whose knowledge is superficial and his reputation among his fellows small; on the other the unrecognised pioneer, whose writings are eagerly read and whose wards and operating theatre are thronged with visitors, but whose consulting-room is empty.

William Heneage Ogilvie, 1887-1971

12   American surgery is like American football; they run about like hell for 10 minutes, and then stop and have a huddle.

William Heneage Ogilvie, 1887-1971

13   Operating as a sport is a purely British conception, and its home is the cottage hospital.

William Heneage Ogilvie, 1887-1971

14   Surgery; like statecraft, requires an international headquarters, like the League of Nations ... where all new discoveries would be demonstrated and all records filed.

William Heneage Ogilvie, 1887-1971

15   On the continent the system of large professorial clinics, where the word of one man is law over decades, while assistants grow old and fixed in his service, tends to the perpetuation of local tradition and the cramping of true originality as against mere showmanship.

William Heneage Ogilvie, 1887-1971

16   In America ... the orthodoxy of past generations is often wrongly condemned on insufficient grounds; treatment is largely a matter of fashion, and each innovation is accepted as an advance, till a newer method displaces it.

William Heneage Ogilvie, 1887-1971

17   German surgery is based on the laboratory and operating theatre, but rarely approaches the bedside; it produces superb surgical pathologists and brilliant operators, but few clinicians or clinical teachers of any importance.

William Heneage Ogilvie, 1887-1971

18   If one were to generalize at all, one might say that the surgery of Germany, on the whole, has a tendency to be radical, that of England conservative, France, brilliant but provincial.

Owen H Wangensteen, 1898-1981

19   It would be easy for me to free myself from being classified as Jew; I could point out that I am only partially of Jewish descent. But by doing so I would declare my inherited Jewish heritage as mediocre. But in reality, I am very proud to possess the blood of a race which for thousands of years has definitively enriched the culture of practically all countries in spite of evil physical and spiritual persecutions.

Rudolf Nissen, 1896-1981

20   The whole affair ... was an interesting study in the formation of medical opinion, showing the way in which truth gets overlaid by muddled thinking, and how exaggerated deference is paid to a given opinion because it emanates from a large American clinic rather than from a smaller London one.

Geoffrey Keynes, 1887-1982

21   Our system remains peculiarly American, free of the undemocratic geheimrat system that has permeated Europe or the unstructured laissez faire preceptorial system of the United Kingdom.

Alexander J Walt, 1923-1996

22   Don't worry about limited knowledge of English; what keeps me awake at night are surgeons with limited surgery!

Ravindra Padmanabhan, 1950-2001

23 If an American doctor wants to double his income, he doubles his fees; if a French doctor wants to double his income, he takes twice as many appendixes.

Lynn Payer, 1945-2001

24 The popularity of coronary bypass surgery concords with the American culture biases of aggressive treatment and with the American view of the body as a machine.

Lynn Payer, 1945-2001

25 There are countries who have ideas, hardly manage the English language, have no oil, and have no trials. There are other countries who have ideas, are artists in surgical techniques, hardly manage the English language, have no oil and no trials. There are still other countries who seldom have ideas, know how to speak English, have oil and controlled clinical trials.

Lynn Payer, 1945-2001

26 In my university time in the USSR we used to joke: optimists learn English, pessimists learn Chinese, realists learn AK-47.

Viatcheslav (Slava) Ryndine

27 It is easier for doctors to reject a foreign study.

Fritz Beller

28 When you see a patient's wound has been treated by a Spanish doctor, it will have two sutures, since in Spain doctors are paid by treating the wound. An Austrian doctor would have put in six sutures, and a Belgian doctor would have put in as many sutures as he could, as they are paid by the number of sutures.

Henk Lamberts

29 The moral of all this could be summed up as: if you have low standard medical schools as in Italy, it makes no difference to have a surgeon who deserves almost a standing ovation at a meeting such as the last ACS; at the end even important people such as the Pope will benefit from the products of this culture.

Melchiorre Costa

It is less dangerous

to leap from the

Clifton Suspension

Bridge than to suffer

from acute intestinal

obstruction and

decline operation.

Fredrick Treves,

1853-1923

Chapter 49

Intestine

1   The jejunum is more exempt from morbid conditions than any other portion of the alimentary canal.
William Withey Gull, 1816-1890

2   When thou examinest the obstruction in his abdomen and thou findest that he is not in a condition to leap the Nile, his stomach is swollen and his chest asthmatic, then say thou to him: it is the blood that has got itself fixed and does not circulate.
George Ebers, 1837-1898, surgical papyrus

3   It is less dangerous to leap from the Clifton Suspension Bridge than to suffer from acute intestinal obstruction and decline operation.
Fredrick Treves, 1853-1923

4   The frequent necessity of resection for the relief of intestinal obstruction is a sombre commentary on the diagnostic ability of the profession. In the very large majority of cases delay is responsible rather than the primary cause of ileus.

William J Mayo, 1861-1939

5   My work essentially has been that of plumber of the alimentary canal. I have worked on both ends, but largely in between.

Owen H Wangensteen, 1898-1981

6   Lysis of all small bowel adhesions is not required because I believe that the bowel is "locked in the open position" by these chronic adhesions.

Timothy Fabian

7   I hav finally kum to the konklusion that a good reliable sett ov bowels iz wurth more tu a man, than enny quantity of brains.

8   Never let the sun set or the dawn rise over a complete intestinal obstruction.

From the editor

◆ The only thing predictable about small bowel obstruction is its unpredictability.

◆ It is almost impossible to further increase the current mortality associated with acute mesenteric ischemia.

I firmly believe

that the best

possible operation

is not the same

thing as the best

operation possible.

Rodney Smith,

1914-1998

Chapter 50

Judgment

1   Life is short and art is long; the crisis is fleeting, experience risky, decision difficult.
Hippocrates, 460-377 BC

2   The experienced doctor will take care not to aggravate the sick person's malady by tiring but injurious efforts.
Hermann Boerhaave, 1668-1738

3   When you come to be an operator, you would do well to catechise yourself: does the operation bid fair to give relief? Is it to be of advantage, as promoting the improvement of the profession? Has self any thing to do with the matter - vanity of display, or personal distinction and consequent emolument?
Benjamin Bell, 1749-1806

4   In the performance of our duty one feeling should direct us; the case we should consider as our own, and we should ask

ourselves, whether, placed under similar circumstances, we should choose to submit to the pain and danger we are about to inflict.

Astley Paston Cooper, 1768-1841

5   If we go into a court of law, we see the bench occupied by the learned judges ... and a jury ... what are they met to decide? Perhaps a matter of money or succession. Even if it should be a criminal court, what a contrast have we with the situation of a surgeon on whose single decision the life of a fellow creature depends... The surgeon cannot lean upon the judgment of others... He has to examine all the evidence, often strangely perverted; he must judge, unaided by friendly counsel... a thing of the greatest difficulty.

Charles Bell, 1774-1842

6   Shakiness of the hand may be some bar to the successful performance of an operation, but he of a shaky mind is hopeless.

William Macewen, 1848-1924

7   In deciding question, he should be unswerved by sympathy, unlured by gain, unterrified by censure.

J Chalmers Da Costa, 1863-1933

8   The physician is obligated to consider more than a diseased organ, more even than the whole man - he must view the man in his world.

Harvey Williams Cushing, 1869-1939

9   Judgement is a great asset; it makes the diagnostician and surgeon both supermen.

Charles H Mayo, 1865-1939

10   I never say of an operation that it is without danger.

August Bier, 1861-1949

11   A problem of baffling simplicity.

Lockhart-Mummerys, 1875-?

12   When the judgement of the surgeon shows that operation is clearly indicated, there are three outstanding features the protection of the patient demands: conservatism strictly consistent with efficiency; simplicity of technique restricted to what is absolutely necessary; operative skills, including genteelness, manipulative dexterity and careful speed.

Max Thorek, 1880-1960

13   Surgical judgement is the crowning attribute of a great surgeon since it is always acquired, with much labour and over a long time, yet, when acquired, it can be shared with and to some extent imparted to others who are prepared to subject themselves to a similar discipline. Judgement means the making of right decisions.

William Heneage Ogilvie, 1887-1971

14   Poor judgment is responsible for much bad surgery, including the withholding of operations that are necessary or advisable, the performance of unnecessary and superfluous operations, and the performance of inefficient, imperfect, and wrongly chosen ones.

Charles FM Saint, 1886-1973

15   If you are not sure, it isn't.

Mark M Ravitch, 1910-1989

16   Judgment moderates the response to recognized categories.

Charles M Abernathy, 1941-1994

17   I firmly believe that the best possible operation is not the same thing as the best operation possible.

Rodney Smith, 1914-1998

18   A surgeon maintains a mental catalogue of the things he did wrong at various times in his career and tries never to repeat them.

Francis D Moore, 1913-2001

19   Are you sure that you are the best person for the job?

Francis D Moore, 1913-2001

20   My personal thesis is that surgical judgment should be based on "numbers", with the caveat that the numbers themselves may be suspect.

Seymour I Schwartz

21   The truth is that surgical decision-making is based on the marriage of evidence from clinical studies, inferences from biology, and the elusive element of surgical experience.

John Marshall

22   Never admit elective cases straight from the outpatient department.

Flavio Frigo

23   Do more for the high risk and less for the low risk.

Ron Nichols

24   Never offer a patient an operation you wouldn't offer to your mother.

25   The Everest Syndrome: just because you can climb a mountain does not mean that you have to climb it; the same is true for any operation.

26   Anything in surgery boils down to risk and benefit.

27   Let someone else kill the patient - do not be a hero.

28   We diagnose only things we think about; we think only about things that we have studied.

29   The operation should be tailored to the patient not vice versa.

30   Re-visit the Mecca which produced you; you'll be surprised that what you consider a holy grail has become anachronistic.

31   Some surgeons are often wrong, but never in doubt.

32   Believe half of what you see and nothing of what you hear.

33   90% of what I'll be telling you is true; it's your job to figure out what, in what I say, represents the other 10%.

34   Don't throw away all the wisdom you have because of the last case you have seen.

35   Believe nobody - question everything.

36   It is more difficult to decide when not to operate than when to operate and what operation to perform.

37   No amount of genius can overcome a preoccupation with detail.

38   It is preferable to use superior judgment to avoid having to use superior skill.

From the editor

♦ "Big" operation in "fit" patients may be "small". "Small" operation in sick patients may be "big". A "big" surgeon knows to tailor the operation and its trauma to the patient and his disease.

♦ For elective and benign conditions always let the patient convince you that the planned operation is indicated.

♦ There are a few ways to skin a cat - the simplest is usually the best.

Chapter 51

Laparoscopy

1   There are warnings all around us - the flexible colonoscope led to a growth of industry of removal of barely visible quasi-polyps. The flexible gastroscope led to repetitive gastroduodenal endoscopic investigation for chronic remunerative gastritis. Minimal-access surgery should not be exploited along similar lines.

Alexander J Walt, 1923-1996

2   Seeing with enlargement is the prerequisite for the success of this new surgical concept. For me, this is the reason minilaparotomy is wrong. It cannot be rescued from its uselessness even using controlled clinical studies.

Hans Troidl

3   Personally I do not know the pioneers of endoscopic surgery well. Many of the pioneers ... are open-minded thinkers, are enthusiastic about their work (even passionate), are hard workers, have other

We are looking at a glass of beer.

Open surgery is the beer; laparoscopy is the foam.

Herand Abcarian

interests, have time to enjoy their lives, have an innocent nature, see the abnormal (the normal probably bores them), and they are venturesome. Their colleagues (the normal people) consider them crazy, exotic, outsiders; they are laughed at, mocked, and even fought.

Hans Troidl

4   We are looking at a glass of beer. Open surgery is the beer; laparoscopy is the foam.

Herand Abcarian

From the editor

◆   The world might look brighter through the (laparoscopic) camera, but not everything bright is gold.

◆   Diagnostic laparoscopy could be viewed as a controlled penetrating abdominal trauma.

Chapter 52

Lecture

Your words

must be as

sharp as the

scalpel you hold.

1   It is the peculiarity of the bore that he is the last person to find himself out.
Oliver Wendell Holmes, 1809-1894

2   Begin with an arresting sentence; close with a strong summary; in between speak simply, clearly, and always to the point; and above all be brief.
William J Mayo, 1861-1939

3   If the crowd outside doesn't shut up, I will stop telling dirty jokes.
J Engelbert Dunphy, 1908-1981

4   Any speech made in public was a work of art, a perfectly coordinated flow of oratory. I had never quite known what the word "oratory" meant until I heard Moynihan producing it. He was very much aware of his gift and all his most impromptu speeches had been carefully rehearsed.
Geoffrey Keynes, 1887-1982

5   Never put more than six lines to a slide.
                                    Robert M Zollinger, 1903-1992

6   A major lecture, oration, or article by custom today is constructed
     with a list, compiled presumably with a computer, of all the
     publications on the subject. One must fit one's own observation into
     a prefabricated structure built around what dozens of authors have
     written about what hundreds of people have said on the subject...
     I do not work this way at all.
                                    Rodney Smith, 1914-1998

7   Your words must be as sharp as the scalpel you hold.

From the editor

◆   All surgeons appear powerful on Power Point; all seem to be graduates of Harvard
     on Harvard Graphics.

Chapter 53

Malpractice & Law

1   If a doctor has treated a man with a metal knife for a severe wound, and has caused the man to die, his hands shall be cut off.
Hammurabi's Code, ~2000 BC

2   The knife is dangerous in the hand of the wise, let alone in the hand of the fool.
Hebrew proverb

3   Not that I am unaware that the wickedness of many of our craft, accompanied by ignorance, is the reason that this part of surgery is so held in contempt.
Pierre Franco, 1500-1561

4   Surgeons who commit indefinite frauds in putting forth their charms and their superstitions, who often spend much time to charm, after which they begin by making an incision but are unable to complete the operation, keeping the poor patient in the meantime, in great languishment.
Pierre Franco, 1500-1561

Doctors are just the same as lawyers; the only difference is that lawyers merely rob you, whereas doctors rob you and kill you, too.

Anton Chekhov,

1860-1904

5   We must all hang together, or we will surely all hang separately.
Thomas Paine, 1737-1809

6   I had to pay two hundred pounds damage, and the law expenses were two hundred pounds more. The loss of the money I did not feel, but I have severely felt being pointed at as an ignorant man.
Astley Paston Cooper, 1768-1841

7   Nor is the public aware of the temptation, which men of our profession withstand. Credit for great abilities, gratitude for services performed, and high emoluments are ready to be bestowed for a little deception, and that obliquity of conduct, which does not amount to actual crime.
Charles Bell, 1774-1842

8   How rarely do our medicines do good? How often do they make our patients really worse! I fearlessly assert that in most cases the sufferer would be safer without a physician than with one. I have seen enough of malpractice of my professional brethren to warrant the strong language I employ.
Francis Hopkins Ramadge, 1793-1867

9   Difficult as it may be to cure, it is always easy to poison and to kill.
Ralph Waldo Emerson, 1803-1882

10   These people say further, that the greater part of the illness, which exists in their country, is brought about by the insane manner in which it is treated.
Samuel Butler, 1835-1902

11   Doctors are just the same as lawyers; the only difference is that lawyers merely rob you, whereas doctors rob you and kill you, too.
Anton Chekhov, 1860-1904

12   I have made a point all my life to mistrust all doctors, lawyers and women. They are shammers and deceivers.
Anton Chekhov, 1860-1904

13   We waste much time blushing for the evil things done by our friends.
J Chalmers Da Costa, 1863-1933

14   Lawyers sue us for the slightest provocation - put us under subpoena even when we know nothing of the case on trial - cross examine us with scorn and with a morbid interest in our private affairs, and combat us when we try to collect a proper fee from a reluctant millionaire.

J Chalmers Da Costa, 1863-1933

15   Every now and then I see a judge on the bench who reminds me of a fly in amber. I know he is there, but I can't imagine how he got there.

J Chalmers Da Costa, 1863-1933

16   Every now and then an expert witness is found to possess one of those well-trained memories which is able to remember everything advantageous and nothing harmful to that side of the case.

J Chalmers Da Costa, 1863-1933

17   Surgery, like aviation, is in itself not inherently dangerous. But to an even greater degree than the sea, it is terribly unforgiving of any carelessness, incapacity, or neglect.

Francis D Moore, 1913-2001

18   Who wants to pay for the dead?

Monte Python

19   Medical practice has also evolved so that now a defensive element tempers the physician's diagnostic and therapeutic approach ... defensive medicine, with its economic and emotional consequences, is a pollutant byproduct of society that should be eradicated.

Seymour I Schwartz

20   As I understand surgeons in the US should follow the standards of care. Then how do you try new techniques - because every new way of treatment is the deviation from standard of care?

Nick Mendel

21   Surgery is the most dangerous activity of legal society.

PO Nyström

22   The case record is written for the public prosecutor.
Youry Vladimirovitch Plotnicov

23   The real problem isn't how to stop bad doctors from harming, even killing, the patients. It's how to prevent good doctors from doing so.
Atul Gawande

24   Risk management begins just when you first meet the patient and family.

25   Acknowledge each member of the family - look into his or her eye - one of them may be the one to initiate the lawsuit against you.

26   If it has not been written it did not exist.

27   The only thing jurors hate more than cocky surgeons are cocky lawyers.

28   Two thirds of the world's lawyers live in the USA.

29   Sins of omission are harder to prove than sins of commission.

From the editor

◆ Malpractice in the setting of public-socialized medicine usually implies that too little was done; malpractice in the setting of a private-capitalistic system usually means that too much has been done; in the public sector the too little is even less at night or weekends while in the private setting the too much is always more during the week and day hours.

◆ If Hammurabi's Code would be in effect today, almost half of the surgeons would go around without arms.

Chapter 54

Military surgery

1   He who wishes to be a surgeon should go to war.

Hippocrates, 460-377 BC

2   Boer War: in this war a man wounded in the abdomen dies if he is operated on and remains alive if he is left in peace.

William MacCormac, 1836-1901

3   The surgeon is not yet born who does not think that he is the one who can close in war a gunshot wound primarily.

Philip Mitchiner, ~1939

4   Good surgery must be done as far forward as possible. If it is too good, in the sense of too elaborately equipped, it will not be far enough forward, and if it is too far forward it will not be good enough.

William Heneage Ogilvie, 1887-1971

He who wishes to be a surgeon should go to war.

Hippocrates,

460-377 BC

5 Today we expect in the injuries of the head, chest and abdomen a recovery rate twice that of the last war ... so satisfactory are the results that we may be in danger of forgetting that we are only helping the tissues to fight the battle at which they are so expert, not fighting it for them.

William Heneage Ogilvie, 1887-1971

6 To the average professional officer, the military doctor is an unwillingly tolerated noncombatant who takes sick call, gives cathartic pills, makes transportation troubles, complicates tactical plans, and causes the water to smell bad.

Hans Zinsser

7 As with most scientific advances made during wartime, the fundamental observations were made during times of peace and relative tranquility. Development of knowledge is hastened and dramatized during war, when sheer numbers of casualties often prompt significant surgical advance.

Ben Eiseman

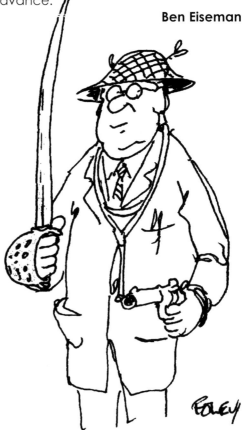

He who wishes to be a surgeon should go to war.

Chapter 55

Money matters

1   A physician who heals for nothing is worth nothing.

The Talmud

2   Doctors cut, burn, and torture the sick, and then demand of them an undeserved fee for such services.

Heraclitus, ~513 BC

3   Sometimes give your services for nothing ... and if there be an opportunity of serving one who is a stranger in financial straits, give full assistance to all such. For where there is love of man, there is also love of the art.

Hippocrates, 460-377 BC

4   Know just this; a remuneration worthy of your labours, that is to say, a very good fee, makes for the authority of the physician and increases the confidence which the patient has in him, even if the physician be of great ignorance.

William of Salicet, 1210-1277

The time during which a surgeon can charge large fees is brief.

J Chalmers Da Costa, 1863-1933

5   He should give advice to the poor for sake of God; he should make the rich pay well if he can.

Henri de Mondeville, 1260-1320

6   He should help the poor according to whatever they are able to pay but should ask good reward from the rich.

Hieronymus Brunschwig, 1450-1512

7   Every man desires to acquire wealth in order that he may give it to the doctors, the destroyers of life; therefore they ought to be rich.

Leonardo da Vinci, 1452-1519

8   He shall also not for the sake of money, undertake the impossible that may do him harm or give him a poor reputation.

Hans von Gersdorff, 1480-1540

9   As long as men are liable to die and are desirous to live, a physician will be made fun of, but he will be well paid.

Jean de La Bruyère, 1645-1696

10   The best patients are the poor because the Lord has taken it upon Himself to pay me for them.

Herman Boerhaave, 1668-1738

11   God heals, and the doctor takes the fees.

Benjamin Franklin, 1706-1790

12   I must go and earn this damned guinea or I shall be sure to want it tomorrow.

John Hunter, 1728-1793

13   Private patients, if they do not like me, can go elsewhere; but the poor devils in the hospital I am bound to take care of.

John Abernethy, 1764-1831

14   Physicians are the natural attorneys of the poor and social problems should largely be solved by them.

Rudolph Virchow, 1821-1902

15   Surgical services have no fixed cost; they are without value in that they are invaluable.

Augustus Charles Bernays, 1854-1907

16   A fashionable surgeon, like a pelican, can be recognized by the size of his bill.

J Chalmers Da Costa, 1863-1933

17   The time during which a surgeon can charge large fees is brief.

J Chalmers Da Costa, 1863-1933

18   As a rule, at the best, a surgeon has twenty five years in which to make and lay by enough to provide for his old age and for the decent support of his family after his death.

J Chalmers Da Costa, 1863-1933

19   A patient who says he must borrow money to pay you will borrow the money, but won't pay you.

J Chalmers Da Costa, 1863-1933

20   A man who pays his surgeon many gleaming compliments seldom pays him anything.

J Chalmers Da Costa, 1863-1933

21   Very few people are able to pay large fees. Very few of those who are able to do so are willing.

J Chalmers Da Costa, 1863-1933

22   In using the term "success" I do not regard it synonymous with wealth. Some men are so busy making money that they have no time to study, to observe, or to think. A rich man who has not brought honor to his profession is not a real success.

J Chalmers Da Costa, 1863-1933

23   It is a man's duty to provide moderately for his family, but anything beyond this may be detrimental to his descendants.

William J Mayo, 1861-1939

24   Commercialism in medicine never leads to true satisfaction, and to maintain our self-respect is more precious than gold.

William J Mayo, 1861-1939

25   Banker: "I don't understand why, with such an income, your account is so frequently overdrawn". Sauerbruch: "if you as a banker don't know, how can I possibly understand it?"

Ernst Ferdinand Sauerbruch, 1875-1951

26   It is asking more than human perfection to assume that a surgeon's judgment may not be influenced unconsciously by pressing financial need.

Edwin P Lehman, 1888-1954

27   Most medical men are amateurs at finance, and what is learned comes through bitter experience.

Harold Gillies, 1882-1960, & Ralph D Millard, Jr.

28   The costs of attempting to provide an indefinitely long life are infinite.

Alexander J Walt, 1923-1996

29   *Mucho trabajo, poko dinero* - Much trouble, little money.

NB Pai, 1937-1999

30   Filled with idealism, students nowadays are plunged into a gaudy and greedy commercial world of corporate profit and personal wealth. They see the huge earnings of insurance companies, hospitals (even the "nonprofits"), administration and doctors. They are not blind to the million-dollar incomes of many physicians and surgeons today, shocking though they may be to us old-timers. Everyone wants to make a buck out of the medical monster. That is why it costs so much to keep it alive.

Francis D Moore, 1913-2001

31   Commercialism and professionalism are parallel streams in our society that can coexist in peace. When they start to get mixed with each other, beware.

Francis D Moore, 1913-2001

32   The hospital is like a shopping mall.

PO Nyström

33   How do you hide $20.00 from an orthopaedic surgeon? Put it in the chart.

Paul M Dubois

How do you hide $20.00 from an anaesthesiologist? Put it in the operating room. How do you hide $20.00 from a plastic surgeon? Impossible, you can't hide money from them.

Victor Bruscagin

34   We are known to the world as a nation of dollar chasers where nearly everything that should control the right of living is sacrificed to the Moloch of money.

CW Oviatt

35   *De dinero y bondad, siempre la mitad* - of money and goodness, always in the middle.

Eric Olivero

36   The salary is not necessary for the good surgeon, he may support himself.

O Blinnicov (From Russian by Youry Vladimirovitch Plotnicov)

37   When money gets tight, people get mean.

Thomas Matthews Haizlip Sr

38   More surgeons live of the disease than people who die from it.

39   The more often you put your finger on an instrument in your office, the less often you will put your foot in your mouth.

40 Exploratory operation: a remunerative reconnaissance.

41 It is the surgeon who benefits most from elective surgery.

42 Negative wallet biopsy=operating on the non-insured.

43 When the patient is ill, surgeon is God; when he is cured, doctor is Man; when he gets the bill, doctor is the Devil.

44 You can be a very rich surgeon or a very good surgeon but rarely both.

From the editor

◆ Unfortunately, many good surgeons earn less than good prostitutes.

Chapter 56

Morbid obesity

1 Patients who are naturally very fat are apt to die earlier than those who are slender.
   Hippocrates, 460-377 BC

2 Obesity is a mental state, a disease brought on by boredom and disappointment.
   Cyril Connolly, 1903-1974

3 Imprisoned in every fat man a thin one is wildly signalling to be let out.
   Cyril Connolly, 1903-1974

4 Do not treat supratentorial conditions with infratentorial procedures.

5 And the Lord said to the surgeon on Judgment Day: I made them fat, you should have left them this way.

It is a certain surgical personality which adopts bariatric surgery as its sole career.

Moshe Schein

The closer you

come to the US

the longer and

redder become the

artificial nails of

the scrub nurses.

Moshe Schein

Chapter 57

Nursing

1 Taking care of such an unhappy patient, with so little prospect of any success, is one of the heaviest loads one can lay on a human being, which only women can carry, for any length of time with never-ending patience.
Theodor Billroth, 1829-1894

2 Let us now remember many honourable women, such as bade us turn again when we were like to die.
Rudyard Kipling, 1865-1936

3 The trained nurse has given nursing the human, or shall we say, the divine touch, and made the hospital desirable for patients with serious ailments regardless of their home advantages.
Charles H Mayo, 1865-1939

4 Every nurse learns that there are moments when it is better to leave a patient alone, because sympathy would only make matters worse.
Harold Gillies, 1882-1960, & Ralph D Millard, Jr.

Chapter 58

Old patients

1   Old have fewer complaints than young; but those chronic diseases which do befall them generally never leave them.
    Hippocrates, 460-377 BC

2   Long ago I leaned from my father to put old people to bed only for as short a time as was absolutely necessary, for they were like a foundered horse; if they got down it was difficult for them to get up, and their strength ebbed away very rapidly while in bed.
    Charles H Mayo, 1865-1939

3   The aged, as we must never forget, are always lonesome ... they belong to the unforgiving past. They are as strangers in the land.
    Alfred Worcester, 1855-1951

4   A German doctor explained this to me once using the card house analogy ... and I see this happen time and again with the super oldies in our ICU. These folks maintain a fragile system quite well ... until it gets disturbed.
    PO Nyström

The aged, as we must never forget, are always lonesome...they belong to the unforgiving past. They are as strangers in the land.

Alfred Worcester, 1855-1951

5 The principles of minimal interference is paramount in the management of the elderly ... the older, more rigid personality is like a crystal easily shattered by unwise impacts.

David Seegal

6 We have to operate soon before he dies of natural causes.

Gail Waldby

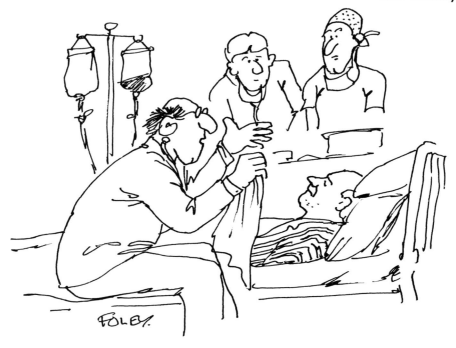

We have to operate soon before he dies of natural causes.

From the editor

◆ Your old patient is like old wine: good vintage allowed him to reach an advanced age. Both are very sensitive to a faulty cork or excessive surgery.

Chapter 59

Old & young surgeons

1   My lamp is almost extinguished. I hope it has burned for benefit of others.
     Percivall Pott, 1714-1788

2   It might ... be of singular advantage to young surgeons, particularly before they begin an operation to go through every part of it attentively in their own minds to consider every possible accident which may happen and to have the proper remedies at hand in case they should; and in all operations of delicacy and difficulty to act with deliberation.
     John Jones, 1729-1791

3   To the students and young parishioners in surgery through all America ... if any of you, by observing the following rules, should save a life, or even a limb of but one civilian ... I shall think myself richly rewarded for my labor.
     John Jones, 1729-1791

4   When I was young, patients were afraid of me; now that I am old, I am afraid of patients.
     Johann Peter Frank, 1745-1821

It is very difficult to slow down. The practice of medicine is like heart muscle contraction - it's all or none.

Béla Schick,

1877-1967

5   Young men kill their patients; old men let them die.

James Gregory, 1753-1821

6   When a man falls into his anecdotage, it is a sign for him to retire.

Benjamin Disraeli, 1804-1881

7   The young man knows the rules, but the old man knows the exceptions ... The young man feels uneasy if he is not continually doing something to stir up his patient's internal arrangements. The old man takes things more quietly, and is much more willing to let well enough alone.

Oliver Wendell Holmes, 1809-1894

8   Many people like their doctors mouldly like their cheese.

Oliver Wendell Holmes, 1809-1894

9   A surgeon can continue to operate as long as his hand is steady and his eye keen. Hand and eye are apt to fail in the sixties.

J Chalmers Da Costa, 1863-1933

10   When a lawyer is about fit to be put on the shelf, he is put on the bench instead. But when the operating surgeon begins to fail, he has to stop.

J Chalmers Da Costa, 1863-1933

11   A young doctor's chief practice is the practice of economy.

J Chalmers Da Costa, 1863-1933

12   Although a doctor may be in the winter of his years, the icicles should never gather in his heart and the lamp of pity should never be extinguished in his soul.

J Chalmers Da Costa, 1863-1933

13   Why not put the surgical age of retirement for the attending surgeon at sixty and the physician at sixty-three or sixty-five, as you think best? I have an idea that the surgeon's fingers are apt to get a little stiff and this makes him less competent before the physician's cerebral vessels do.

Harvey Williams Cushing, 1869-1939

14   The keen clinician, as he grows in experience, becomes more and more valuable as age advances.

William J Mayo, 1861-1939

15   The old should remember that they represent the past, and that the young represent the future.

William J Mayo, 1861-1939

16   Each day as I go through the hospital surrounded by young men, they give me of their dreams and I give them of my expertise, and I get the better of the exchange.

William J Mayo, 1861-1939

17   Longevity is worthwhile only if it prolongs youth rather than old age.

Alexis Carrel, 1873-1944

18   Everything-er-nowadays is too-er-difficult. It is time that the-er-younger men took my-er-place.

Grant Massie, 1896-1964

19   It is very difficult to slow down. The practice of medicine is like heart muscle contraction - it's all or none.

Béla Schick, 1877-1967

20   Every Chief of Service should have a pet dog, like Ulysses had. When he retires from the hospital he should leave his dog on the floor of the department he served, because when he returns the only one who will recognize him will be his dog.

Béla Schick, 1877-1967

21   A physician's life is a constant and losing battle against obsolescence.

Mark M Ravitch, 1910-1989

22   Young surgeons, busy mastering the technicalities of the art, are particularly alert to seize every legitimate opportunity to practise technical manoeuvres, the more complicated the better.

Stanley O Hoerr, 1909-1990

23   A danger of aging is the temptation to look back without looking forward, probably because the latter prospect is so understandably discouraging. I would like to avoid this temporal hang-up.

Alexander J Walt, 1923-1996

24   Hardening of the attitude occurs before hardening of the arteries.

Matt Oliver

25   Beware of the young doctor and old barber.

26   There are bold surgeons and old surgeons but few old-bold surgeons.

27   Surgeons get long lives and short memories.

28   A surgeon should be young, a physician old.

29   Retiring department chairman: in one day he goes from "who's who" to "who's he?"

30   Young surgeons err in believing that knowledge can compensate for lack of experience; old surgeons err in believing that experience can compensate for lack of knowledge.

From the editor ◆ Young surgeons have to learn to relax; to understand that time is the ultimate healer; to let nature deal with the disease. So sit down and relax; do not stand there with your knife always ready to do unnecessary things.

Chapter 60

On call

Everything gets worse at night.

1   Almost everyone who goes to bed counts upon a full night's rest: like a picket at the outposts, the doctor must be ever on call.
Karl Marx, 1796-1877

2   Important decisions often have to be made at night when the physician, weary with the day's work, and with perceptions and reasoning faculties somewhat jabbed, is both physically and mentally below his best.
Zachary Cope, 1881-1974

3   Midnight calls are not made for the sake of hearing the surgeon's voice.
Mark M Ravitch, 1910-1989

4   The progress of disease is not suspended between 5pm and morning rounds.
Mark M Ravitch, 1910-1989

5   If you don't operate on your night on call you'll operate on your night off call.

6   If you stay up all day, you'll stay up all night.

7   Never walk through the ER unless you are called.

8   In the ER when you don't know what's wrong, keep inserting the tubes until someone who knows arrives.

9   If he didn't want an operation why did he come to the ER at this time of night?

10   Everything gets worse at night.

Chapter 61

Operating room

1   If it be a great operation, and especially if the assistant and nurses are not habituated, be careful to appoint them their places and their duties; for nothing tends more to the right performance of an operation of magnitude, than the composure and quietness which results from arrangement.

Benjamin Bell, 1749-1806

2   The hospital, the operating room, and the wards should be laboratories, laboratories of the highest order.

William Stewart Halsted, 1852-1922

3   When results by simple methods in private houses are as good as results by highly complex and expensive processes in hospital operating rooms, the answer as to the justifiability of the simpler methods seems perfectly clear.

J Chalmers Da Costa, 1863-1933

God indeed rewards those who enter the OR with a prepared mind.

Timothy Fabian

4   Gowns are, of course, necessary, as are caps also - to prevent hair and dandruff from falling into the wound; but a face mask, I do not believe to be necessary, if the operator is careful that in talking his face is not near to ... the wound. Of course if he is bearded like the pard, suffers with a hacking catarrh, and sprays into the boundless universe while he talks, then it is imperative that he should wear a mask.

J Chalmers Da Costa, 1863-1933

5   What is sauce for the goose is sauce for the gander. Why should not the surgeon use the gloves as well as the nurse?

Joseph C Bloodgood, 1867-1935

6   The most important person in the operating room is the patient.

Russell John Howard, 1875-1942

7   The opportunity to learn walks with any surgeon who enters the operating room with questions on his mind.

Wilder Penfield, 1891-1976

8   About Thomas P Dunhill (1876-1957): when speaking there was no time to seek out all the right words. A characteristic sentence uttered when under the stress in the operating theatre ran: "tell Miss thing to put the thing in the thing".

Geoffrey Keynes, 1887-1982

9   Our turf - our kingdom - is the operating room, where we are now beginning to feel very secure; for here not only is there a sense of discipline, there is also a pecking order rarely found elsewhere in the hospital. The king, the defender of faith, is the surgeon who does the cutting!

Dominic A DeLaurentis

10   God indeed rewards those who enter the OR with a prepared mind.

Timothy Fabian

11   Never leave the operating room without thanking each member of the team; then go and talk to the family.

Chapter 62

Operating (technical)

1   The things relating to surgery, are the patient; the operator; the assistants; the instruments; the light, where and how; how many things, and how; where the body, and the instruments; the time; the manner; the place.
Hippocrates, 460-377 BC

2   It is well to wax the twisted thread so that it does not cut the flesh.
Jean Yperman, 1260-1310

3   I can recognize a good surgeon, not by how he cuts, but how he sews.
Johan Mikulicz-Radecki, 1850-1905

4   Use as thin a ligature as seems consistent with the required strength.
Augustus Charles Bernays, 1854-1907

5   Not every little artery needs tying; a clamp left on for a few minutes often suffices and avoids a foreign substance in the wound.
Augustus Charles Bernays, 1854-1907

I can recognize a good surgeon, not by how he cuts, but how he sews.

Johan Mikulicz-Radecki, 1850-1905

6   Twisting arteries is just as safe as tying.

Augustus Charles Bernays, 1854-1907

7   If the wound is perfectly dry, and the tissues never permitted to become even stained in blood, the operator unperturbed, may work for hours without fatigue.

William Stewart Halsted, 1852-1922

8   It is wiser to operate well than brilliantly - a superlative degree of the former, and a reasonable degree of the latter should be the surgeon's aim. Probably many lives have been the direct cost of unbalanced operative brilliancy.

Warren Stone Bickham, 1886-1936

9   While the patient is better off in the hands of a timid, painstaking surgeon than in those of a bold, destructive operator, judicious boldness - the boldness that comes from the certainty of knowledge, and the certainty of one's self - is a creditable asset to the possessor.

Warren Stone Bickham, 1886-1936

10   The boldness that comes from ignorance or recklessness cannot be too sweepingly condemned. Timidity is practically always an agony to the operator himself - often an ignorance of surgical pathology, but much more frequently an ignorance of pure anatomy.

Warren Stone Bickham, 1886-1936

11   Carry out the two fundamental surgical requirements: see what you are doing and leave a dry field.

Charles H Mayo, 1865-1939

12   Technical difficulties are rarely insurmountable with practice, ingenuity, and the passage of time.

Elliott Carr Cutler, 1888-1947

13   I have seen another surgeon of excellent repute place the handle of his knife in his mouth for safe-keeping while he was busy tying ligatures.

Thomas S Cullen, 1868-1953

14   The lack of dexterity may account for almost as much post-operative morbidity and post-operative mortality as does lack of knowledge.

Hugh Devine, 1878-1959

15   Actual operative skill cannot be gained by observation, any more than skill in playing the violin can be had by hearing and seeing a virtuoso performing on that instrument.

Allen O Whipple, 1881-1963

16   When tissues must be cut, a knife is probably the best tool to use, and blunt dissection is usually bad surgery.

William Heneage Ogilvie, 1887-1971

17   The simpler the procedure, the better the results.

Charles FM Saint, 1886-1973

18   As apposed to genuine serious surgery are showmanship and exhibitionism. Showmanship is only produced when visitors are present, whereas exhibitionism is entirely independent of who is present and is, consequently, the greater menace, worst when the surgeon indulges in it even when alone, apparently in self adoration.

Charles FM Saint, 1886-1973

19   Medical illustrators are optimists...

Asher Hirshberg

20   Appose it - don't necrose it.

Karen Tobias

21   When swimming with sharks do not thrash in the water and do not drip blood.

Margaret Dunn

22   I believe in the three principles of surgery: hemostasis, asepsis, and elimination of dead space.

Phil Caropreso

23 I believe these principles are important: bloodless and transfusion-free, tension-free, and pain-free surgery.

PO Nyström

24 Rules are for fools.

Bill Heald

25 In Spanish: *la cirurgia de la gallina - una escarvadita, una cagadita.* Operating like a hen: a little dig, a little excrement...

Jose Lucas Ramirez Gil

26 If it looks good, it might work. If it does not look good, it will never work.

William Silen

27 The severe and incapacitating depression that overtakes many surgeons when they are not doing surgery, that is, not cutting.

Dominic A DeLaurentis

28 There is no cavity that cannot be reached with a number 14 needle and a good strong arm.

Samuel Shem

29 The seven P's of any procedure: Proper Prior Planning Prevents Piss Poor Performance.

Steven Tennenberg

30 If you do only routine cases eventually even they will become difficult.

31 A poor workman blames his tool.

32 The enemy of good is better.

33 It is not a dangerous operation: we have never lost a surgeon doing it.

34 It is better to be lucky than good, and the better you are, the luckier you become.

35   When in doubt cut it out.

36   The operation was a success but the patient died.

37   The first cut is the deepest.

38   There are only two things in surgery: cut and sew.

39   Cut well, sew well, do well...

40   With a knife, pair of scissors, a few clamps, a few fingers and a suture, you can do anything.

41   The index finger is still the best instrument.

42   To any operative video you watch add a pint of blood and sweat; then you'll get the reality.

43   Do not always blame the light.

44   When it's an emergency, it is too late.

45   Cold steel is the best deal.

46   It will never get better if you keep picking at it!

47   Don't look for things that you don't want to find.

48   Not all that is technically feasible is in the patient's best interest.

Internists know

everything but do

nothing; surgeons

know nothing but

do everything;

pathologists know

and do everything,

but too late.

Chapter 63

Other disciplines

1   Only the union of medicine and surgery constitutes the complete doctor.
Sushruta <8th century, BC

2   And even in the cases when we count most on medications, it is evident not only that they often fail to restore health, but that health often returns without them. Whereas in the surgical branch of medicine, one can see that every successful cure ... is due primarily to the manual treatment.
Celsus, 25BC-AD50

3   Internists are seldom jealous of surgeons; nay, they back up and recommend one another.
Plutarch, 46-120

4   Oh Lord, why is there so great a difference between a surgeon and a physician? But thou shalt know well this, that he is no good physician that knows nothing of surgery. And the contrary thereof, a man may be no good surgeon if he knows no physic.
Lanfranc of Milan, ~1315

5   Internal medicine and surgery are based on philosophy and must not be separated except in practice; every physician must be a doctor of both medicines.

Paracelsus, 1493-1541

6   Surgery should with good reason be preferred to pharmacy, since chance contributes much to this part of medicine which deals with drugs; and by contrast, the effects of operations are clearly evident, obvious and certain.

Hieronymus Fabricius ab Aquapendente, 1533-1620

7   Pathologists and radiographers, like surgeons, are liable to error. Their reports should be confirmed by clinical observation.

James Berry, 1860-1946

8   The practice of medicine is a thinker's art, the practice of surgery a plumber's.

Martin H Fischer, 1879-1962

9   The surgeon is sometimes despised by the intelligentsia of medicine as a mechanical craftsman. But though he be a hewer of wood and a drawer of water, he has the assurance that such skills are useful to mankind.

William Heneage Ogilvie, 1887-1971

10   Physicians vary in their attitude to surgery. Some regard the avoidance of an operation as an end in itself, and this may not be really in the patient's interest.

Geoffrey Keynes, 1887-1982

11   An internist whose surgeon acts as the motor end organ to the physician's cerebral cortex, associates with an inadequate surgeon.

Mark M Ravitch, 1910-1989

12   I've always said that the most useful equipment for a successful surgeon is a pessimistic pathologist.

John Rowan Wilson, 1919-?

13   There's nothing in the world more dangerous than an Internal Medicine Resident with a needle in his/her hands.

M Botero

14   What is the heart to an orthopedic surgeon? The organ that pumps cefazolin to the rest of the body.

Michael Châtenay

15   What's the difference between an orthopaedic surgeon and a rhinoceros? One is big and noisy and charges a lot and the other lives in Africa!

16   One CT scan is worth a thousand neurologists.

17   Ask any surgeon: what is the definition of "shifting dullness?" Answer: "rounds in Internal Medicine".

18   Orthopedic surgeon: if you can't pin it or cast it, then screw it.

19   How many cardiothoracic surgeons does it take to screw in a light bulb? One - he just holds up the bulb and the world revolves around him.

20   The only difference between psychiatrists and their patients is that the patients have a chance of getting better.

21   Dermatology is the only specialty in medicine where there are 200 diseases and only three types of cream to treat them.

22   A dermatologist is a doctor who will tell you in Latin what you just told him in your own language.

23   The two underlying principles of dermatology: if it is wet then dry it, if it is dry then wet it.

24   A well-known story: an internist, a pathologist and a surgeon went on a hike, during which they observed a strange bird flying above. The internist looked at the bird through his binocular: "a most peculiar bird, he observed, I wish I could examine it". The pathologist counted all possible species the bird could belong to. The surgeon simply aimed his hunting gun and shot the bird down: "here you are gentlemen, now you may reach your diagnosis".

25   Internists know everything but do nothing; surgeons know nothing but do everything; pathologists know and do everything, but too late.

26   Nothing is more ugly than a code in the radiology suite.

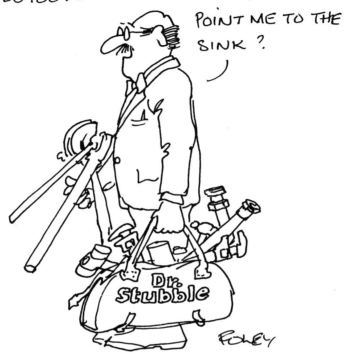

The practice of medicine is a thinker's art, the practice of surgery a plumber's.

From the editor

◆ When an internist wants you to urgently operate on his patient with inflammatory bowel disease, assume that the operation was indicated at least a week ago.

◆ Have you ever seen a gynecologist who is convinced that the "acute abdomen" is gynecological in origin, and not due to acute appendicitis?

◆ Urological and orthopedic wards are a cemetery for patients with a ruptured AAA.

Those who do not

feel pain seldom

think that it is

felt.

Samuel Johnson,

1709-1784

Chapter 64

Pain

---

1   Of two pains occurring together, not in the same part of the body, the stronger weakens the other.

Hippocrates, 460-377 BC

2   We are more sensitive of one little touch of a surgeon's lancet than of twenty wounds with a sword in the heat of fight.

Micheal de Montaigne, 1533-1592

3   The mind is seldom quickened to very vigorous operations but by pain, or the dread of pain.

Samuel Johnson, 1709-1784

4   Those who do not feel pain seldom think that it is felt.

Samuel Johnson, 1709-1784

5   We must all die. But that I can save him from days of torture, that is what I feel as my great and ever new privilege. Pain is a more terrible lord of mankind than even death itself.

Albert Schweitzer, 1875-1965

6   Morphine is the best pain reliever.

Mark M Ravitch, 1910-1989

7   Surgery for poorly specified abdominal pain will always result in permanent abdominal pain.

Clifton K Meador

8   Only a living flesh is painful.

Boris Savchuk

From the editor

◆   The one who operates for pain gets pain.

The time of the

procedure will

vary from 3.5 to 5

hours.

Allan O Whipple,

1881-1963

Chapter 65

Pancreas

1   The pancreas situated high up in the abdominal cavity, and hidden behind such important organs as ... is the least accessible of all abdominal organs, and on this account its affections, wrapped in obscurity, have for the most part constituted subjects for empirical medications.

Nicholas Senn, 1844-1908

2   Acute pancreatitis is the most terrible of all the calamities that occur in connection with the abdominal viscera.

Berkeley Moynihan, 1865-1936

3   The time of the procedure will vary from 3.5 to 5 hours.

Allan O Whipple, 1881-1963

4   To this internist before performing the first total pancreatectomy: "will you promise to keep the patient alive if I remove her entire pancreas?"

James T Priestly, ~1979

5 For pancreatic trauma: treat the pancreas like a crawfish, suck the head ... eat the tail.

Timothy Fabian

6 Do not treat severe acute pancreatitis with daily CT scans.

Sai Sajja

7 Eat whenever you can and pee whenever you can because you never know when you'll get another chance; f*** whenever you can - but don't ever f*** with the pancreas.

Stephen Smith

8 Surgeon, remember that the pancreas is not your friend.

9 God put the pancreas in the back because he did not want surgeons messing with it.

From the editor

◆ Acute necrotizing pancreatitis: during the early phases of the disease "our patience will achieve more than our force" (Edmund Burke. 1820-1895); later on, when called to operate on necrotic and infected complications, remember that "patience and diligence, like faith, remove mountains" (William Penn).

The microscope

does not lie.

Mark M Ravitch,

1910-1989

Chapter 66

Pathology & Physiology

1   There is a most intimate interdependence of physiology, pathology and surgery. Without progress in physiology and pathology, surgery could advance but little, and surgery has paid its debt by contributing much to the knowledge of the pathologist and physiologist, never more than at the present.

William Stewart Halsted, 1852-1922

2   The microscope does not lie.

Mark M Ravitch, 1910-1989

3   Every operation is an experiment in physiology.

Tid Kommer

From the editor

◆   In surgery physiology is the king, anatomy the queen; you can be the prince, but only provided you have the judgment.

◆   When physiology is disrupted attempts at restoring anatomy are futile.

Chapter 67

Patients

1   He should have no familiarity with laymen. For lay people are always wont to malign physicians, and too great a familiarity engenders slander.
William of Salicet, 1210-1277

2   Let the surgeon take care to regulate the whole regimen of the patient's life for joy and happiness. The surgeon must forbid anger, hatred and sadness in the patient. Remind him that the body grows fat from joy, thin from sadness.
Henri de Mondeville, 1260-1320

3   The patient is always more anxious to talk than to listen.
Theodor Billroth, 1829-1894

4   The patient longs for the doctor's daily visit; it is the event upon which all his thoughts and emotions turn.
Theodor Billroth, 1829-1894

The secret for caring for the patient is caring for the patient.

Francis W Peabody, 1881-1927

5   Never believe what a patient tells you his doctor has said.
William Jenner, 1815-1898

6   The patient recovered despite being treated by the best doctors in town.
Leo Tolstoy, 1828-1910

7   A sick person needs someone to trust, and would hold onto a straw, if he senses that he is drowning.
Vinzenz von Czerny, 1842-1916

8   The secret for caring for the patient is caring for the patient.
Francis W Peabody, 1881-1927

9   The treatment of a disease may be entirely impersonal; the care of a patient must be completely personal.
Francis W Peabody, 1881-1927

10   Few things make me more unhappy than ingratitude - ingratitude of patients I have really served, ingratitude of assistants I have really helped.
J Chalmers Da Costa, 1863-1933

11   You can judge some patients by their doctors and some doctors by their patients.
J Chalmers Da Costa, 1863-1933

12   For us an operation is an incident in the day's work, but for our patients it may be, and no doubt it often is, the sternest and most dreaded of all trials, for the mysteries of life and death surround it, and it must be faced alone.
Berkeley Moynihan, 1865-1936

13   It must be remembered that physicians of today are trained to treat the sick, and they must learn how to examine so-called well persons to prevent them from getting sick.
Charles H Mayo, 1865-1939

14   No one in medicine can escape from the satisfaction which goes with grateful patients ... herein ... lies the satisfaction of the practice of medicine and no person in academic life in any of the clinical branches of medicine can succeed who does not respond to such human instincts.

Elliot Carr Cutler, 1888-1947

15   We do not go to the operating table as we go to the theatre, to the picture gallery, to the concert room, to be entertained and delighted; we go to be tormented and maimed, lest a worse thing should befall us .... The experts on whose assurance we face this horror and suffer this mutilation should have no interests but our own to think of; should judge our cases scientifically; and should feel about them kindly.

George Bernard Shaw, 1856-1950

16   The adult can safely be treated as a child, but the converse can lead to disasters.

Lancelot Barrington-Ward, 1884-1953

17   The patient's family will never forgive a guarantee of cure that failed and the patient will not let the physician forget a pronouncement of incurability if he is so fortunate as to survive.

George T Pack, 1898-1969

18   Every patient had become a "case". Not an individual, whereas in fact there was a good reason for regarding each patient as a separate problem for careful consideration according to individual circumstances. I have ever since that time tried to eliminate the word "case" from the writings. It had become a universal curse to medical thinking and still is.

Geoffrey Keynes, 1887-1982

19   No patient is too sick to have his life saved.

Mark M Ravitch, 1910-1989

20   Patients cannot tell their symptoms to the surgeon who will not talk to them.

Mark M Ravitch, 1910-1989

21 Great intelligence, and high position in a patient, bear no relation to his understanding of medical problems.

Mark M Ravitch, 1910-1989

22 When the patient enjoys the surgeon's visit, seeks his touch and his care, and rests secure in trust, a sort of stress-free basal state is established.

Francis D Moore, 1913-2001

23 Nudge the patient - do not kick. Just remember, he's quite sick.

Francis D Moore, 1913-2001

24 Surgery is an irrevocably invasive remedy which links patient and surgeon more clearly than in other areas of medicine.

Charles L Borsk

25 There is among doctors, in acute hospitals at least, a presumption of stupidity in their patients.

Oliver Sacks

26 First thing about being a patient - you have to learn patience.

Oliver Sacks

27 About a patient: it seems to me that his two choices were: 1. Die sooner and wish he had lived longer (no re-operation). 2. Live longer and wish he had died sooner (radical surgery).

Mark Pleatman

28 Who, sir, exactly, were you getting prepared - the patient or yourself?

Frank C Spencer

29 Fit the operation to your patient, not your patient to the operation.

JMT Finney

30   We are rapidly becoming a nation of scars.

Lucy Waite

31   With seriously or terminally ill patients, be wary of kin from afar. They are often trouble.

Clifton K Meador

32   You are the patient's advocate. You work for no one else.

Clifton K Meador

33   Elder female patients with colored hair seldom die.

Julian E Losanoff

34   It's not the surgeon who takes the chance; it's the patient.

Gail Waldby

35   If a patient is an evil person he's going to be safe.

Julian E Losanoff

36   Most patients will survive the surgeon´s shortcomings but some will not.

PO Nyström

37   Encourage difficult patients or families to seek a second opinion.

38   The patient who has bad vibes before the operation is usually right.

39   When it comes to operation, you advise and the patient decides.

40   If you tell a patient to lie on his back he will most likely lie on his stomach.

41   An alcoholic patient is one who drinks more than his surgeon.

42   Do not perform elective surgery on patients you dislike - refer them.

43   Be wary of patients whose risk exceeds their ejection fraction.

From the editor

◆ What the family will decide depends entirely on what and how you'll tell them.

◆ Make the patient earn the operation.

◆ Some patients like to die only after having a few operations.

◆ We tend to remember best those patients we almost killed; we never forget those we actually managed to kill.

Chapter 68

Politics

1   Beware of becoming a "drummer". Don't attend little country or district societies - let the country doctors attend the big meeting. It will be more profitable to them.
Augustus Charles Bernays, 1854-1907

2   If you want to be on the staff of a hospital, lad, pretend you're a fool till you're on it.
Lloyd Roberts, 1853-1920

3   I'll take it up on one condition - that you do not ask other surgeons to co-operate. I am not a co-operator.
William Macewen, 1848-1924

4   The problems of today are our own. Devised to us by the teeming, pushing, often scrambling world we were born into, without our knowledge or consent, and we ourselves must solve them, often in fear and trembling, but always with truth, valour and clean conscience.
Bacon Saunders, 1855-1925

The American Surgical Association (ASA) has talent, the American College of Surgery (ACS) has both talent and muscle, but the American Medical Association (AMA) has access to the voters.

James D Hardy

5   Sometimes when a doctor becomes too lazy to work he becomes a politician.

J Chalmers Da Costa, 1863-1933

6   In some hospitals there is a certain evil tendency ... that ... may be called "the system". It means that certain medical men improperly and unjustly acquire supreme power for selfish interests and not for the public welfare ... some of the staff get more than they deserve and most get less than they need. Those who speak the truth are regarded with fear and aversion. Abuses accumulate. Ignorant neglect is tolerated in some, the best effort is censored in others.

J Chalmers Da Costa, 1863-1933

7   One of the highest functions of a Board of managers of a hospital is to lure, ensnare and capture the shy and predatory rich. Every hospital and college is on the look-out for malefactors of great wealth.

J Chalmers Da Costa, 1863-1933

8   There are few more humiliating things than to see a capable and intelligent physician bowing and scraping to some miserable lunkhead millionaire who holds the strong hand of influence in the community.

J Chalmers Da Costa, 1863-1933

9   About Rudolf Nissen: the fact that that society is the only one to which Nissen belongs may be significant with regard to his practice. I am not aware of the fact that he is doing any thoracic surgery. If he were doing much and were above any criticism he would certainly be a member of the American Association of Thoracic Surgery.

Evarts Ambrose Graham, 1883-1957

10   You are a nobody in surgery unless you have at least as many enemies as friends.

Karl Schein, 1911-1974

11   The feeling that the chairman isn't doing a satisfactory job in any of his several tasks is often shared by his dean, hospital doctors, patients, students, house staff, faculty, research fellows, spouses and children.

E Braunwald

12   The American Surgical Association (ASA) has talent, the American College of Surgery (ACS) has both talent and muscle, but the American Medical Association (AMA) has access to the voters.

James D Hardy

13   One reason why academic conflicts are so brutal is because the stakes are so low.

Arthur E Baue

14   Try to change and keep up but politically it can be suicide to be up to date.

Phil Peverada

15   It is poor judgment to take on the Dean, no matter how poorly he seems to be functioning ... far better to wait for the next turnover of deans.

Isidore Cohn, Jr

16   If you want to be seen you must stand up. If you want to be respected you must sit down.

From the editor

◆ Absolute political correctness suits administrators but not surgeons. It is a recipe for mediocrity. It is pretending to be what we are not.

Do not crucify your patient in a horizontal position.

John R Border,

1926-1996

Chapter 69

Post-operative care

1 The sooner the patient can be removed from the depressing influence of general hospital life the more rapid their convalescence.

Charles H Mayo, 1865-1939

2 Fluids given intravenously bypass all the defenses set up by the body to protect itself against excess of any constituent, against bacterial entry ... they give the patient what the surgeon thinks his tissues need and what they are damned well going to get.

William Heneage Ogilvie, 1887-1971

3 A good heart and kidneys can survive all but the most willfully incompetent fluid regimen.

Mark M Ravitch, 1910-1989

4 Do not crucify your patient in a horizontal position.

John R Border, 1926-1996

5   It cannot be too often emphasized, however, that the post-operative treatment is as essential as the operation, and the surgeon is as much responsible for the post-operative treatment as for the operation.

Roscoe C Giles

6   If renal functions are OK you can administer Coca Cola IV.

Bernard ("Bokki") Rabinowitz

7   Do not risk a cure traded off for a shorter convalescence.

Angus Maciver

8   Post-operatively, no news is good news.

From the editor

◆   The post-operative fart is the best music to the surgeon's ears.

You have to be careful not to become involved in too many small things and not enough big things.

Warren H Cole,

1898-1991

Chapter 70

Practice

1   All practice is theory; all surgery is practice; ergo, all surgery is theory.
Lanfranc of Milan, ~1315

2   What success I have had in my private practice, I have kept no account of, because I had no intention to publish it, that not being sufficiently witnessed.
William Cheselden, 1688-1752

3   The days of waiting for practice are very hard and very dangerous. Those days may make a man or mar him. The same wind which blows out the penny dip urges the flames of the forest fire. Those days go far in determining what sort of man he is and is to be.
J Chalmers Da Costa, 1863-1933

4   There is a grave danger in those waiting hours, those dark hours of poverty and non-recognition. A sensitive soul will shrink, falter

and probably fail. Brooding discontent is apt to dominate and it is a deadly peril. Jealousy may spring up, envy may attain rank luxuriance, bitterness may grow, selfishness, avarice, disloyalty, mental dishonesty may be planted. Low ideas are ever knocking for admission. From them come admiration for despicable things, desires for unworthy objects, and improper professional conduct.

J Chalmers Da Costa, 1863-1933

5   Tact is a valuable attribute in gaining practice. It consists of telling a squint-eyed man that he has a fine, firm chin.

J Chalmers Da Costa, 1863-1933

6   I have never been busy, merely occupied.

Berkeley Moynihan, 1865-1936

7   Three fifths of the practice of medicine depends on common sense, a knowledge of people and human reactions. More than half of the remainder is technological and mechanical, the work of those medically trained artisans we call surgeons.

Harvey Williams Cushing, 1869-1939

8   You have to be careful not to become involved in too many small things and not enough big things.

Warren H Cole, 1898-1991

9   Continuity of care: in surgery, like in chess - you touch, you go.

Danny Rosin

10   Why am I still doing this? Because, doctor, you're too young to retire and too old for a paper route; beside, you don't know how to do anything else.

Bruce J Brener

11   It is incumbent on those of us in the public sector to ensure that services for the poor do not become poor services.

Thomas Matthews Haizlip Sr

12   Surgical conventions are the place where surgeons swap lies about how great their practices are.

13   When the hospital's janitors come to you with their hernias your practice is well established.

14   Aim at a rate of operative cases/meetings of greater than 1.

15   Your job is to satisfy the patient - not the referring MD.

From the editor

◆   The quality of care is in reverse proportion to the volume of paperwork forced by the system on its surgeons.

Chapter 71

Progress

1   A great hypothesis is not the usual path for the advancement of medical knowledge. As a rule, first comes a new or improved method whose application to a variety of problems sometimes leads unexpectedly to greater understanding.

Frank Kittredge Paddock, 1841-1901

2   Those who learned from a great master must surely not be content to imitate his methods, but rather must strive to capture his authentic spirit, and in that spirit seek for new roads.

Berkeley Moynihan, 1865-1936

3   The craft of surgery has in truth nearly reached its limit in respect both of range and safety.

Berkeley Moynihan, 1865-1936

4   Thus the surgeons for each period must discuss the subject and clarify it for themselves, since human experience, which affords opportunity for progress, can be passed on only to a limited extent.

Charles H Mayo, 1865-1939

If you don't like the way surgery is practised today. Just wait a while - it will change.

5   The progress which medicine has made has been due, one sometimes sadly thinks, to the simple fact that ideas are harder to kill than men. The martyr is destroyed, but his faith lives on ... unrecorded on any page ... must always be those ideas that did not survive, life-giving discoveries once almost brought to light and then forced back into darkness to await rediscovery. This is the worst waste our profession encourages.

Max Thorek, 1880-1960

6   We shall not scorn what was done yesterday because we have something better today any more than our interest in the past will cause us to continue the practice of the past.

William Wayne Babcock, 1872-1963

7   Never be the first but never be the last to accept change.

Angus B McLachlin, 1908-1987

8   If you don't like the way surgery is practised today, just wait a while - it will change.

From the editor

◆ The real problem with medical advances is that they are practised indiscriminately.

Chapter 72

Quality of life

1   On brain tumors: we should operate in all cases of tumor for the sake of the relief it affords, even should it be found during the operation that cure by removal is impossible.

Victor Horsley, 1857-1916

2   The surgeon's life is a very hard one. It is a life of endless strain. During most of the hours of every day his faculties are keyed up tense almost to the breaking point, and physical tire goes hand in hand with mental exhaustion.

J Chalmers Da Costa, 1863-1933

3   Withdrawal gives opportunity for a man to develop powers within himself which otherwise may remain dormant in a life crowded with the pursuit of limited objectives.

Edward D Churchill, 1895-1972

Life has meaning (depth) as well as length; quality of life is its second dimension.

Ben Eiseman

4   The quality of survival is as much the surgeon's responsibility as the fact of survival.

Mark M Ravitch, 1910-1989

5   It is difficult to make the asymptomatic patient feel better.

Stanley O Hoerr, 1909-1990

6   Life has meaning (depth) as well as length; quality of life is its second dimension.

Ben Eiseman

7   It is simply not enough for surgeons to aim at the three traditional, easily measurable parameters: operative mortality and morbidity (which we try to reduce) and long-term survival (which we attempt to increase). They must raise their sight to include aspects of quality of life.

Michael Trede

8   A palliative operation should palliate the patient, not the surgeon.

9   Try to leave home in a good mood before major surgery.

10   Do not take your surgical problems home or bring your home to surgery.

From the editor

◆   That "it would have bled" or "would have obstructed" is not an indication for palliative surgery.

◆   A non-nagging wife is an invaluable asset to any surgical career.

Chapter 73

Reading

1   But to become distinguished, nay, to become even respectable in your profession, you must be something more than readers, you must become active thinkers and sifters of knowledge, learn, as Bacon counsels, to weigh and consider books.

Jacob M Da Costa, 1833-1900

2   It is astonishing with how little reading a doctor can practise medicine, but it is not astonishing how badly he may do it.

William Osler, 1849-1919

3   How much better it is to have the walls covered with books with which we are establishing friendly relations, than with pictures of passing interest which we have happened to obtain. Eventually pictures may lose their interest, whereas books never lose their fascination.

William J Mayo, 1861-1939

A real surgeon

reads a book

on a flight - not

a laptop.

Moshe Schein

4　Textbooks of a previous generation were as large as the textbooks of today, but contained a different body of misinformation.

Mark M Ravitch, 1910-1989

5　If you would read more you would invent and discover less.

Karl Sternberg

Chapter 74

Re-operation

1. A surgeon ... is like the skipper of an ocean-going racing yacht. He knows the port he must make, but he cannot foresee the course of the journey. At every stage he must have a plan, based on a working knowledge of his present position, that will allow him to make for the best of several available harbours should things go wrong, or if none is suitable he must know where to find temporary refuge under the lee of the land till he can resume his journey.

   William Heneage Ogilvie, 1887-1971

2. The last man to see the necessity for re-operation is the man who performed the operation.

   Mark M Ravitch, 1910-1989

3. A negative re-laparotomy is better than a positive autopsy but is not, nevertheless, a benign procedure.

   Roger Saadia

The last man to see the necessity for re-operation is the man who performed the operation.

Mark M Ravitch,

1910-1989

4   In re-operative surgery, timing is everything.

Timothy Fabian

5   It's better to save a patient in two operations than killing him in one.

Hernan Diaz

6   This guy is too sick not to be re-operated upon.

◆ Early re-operation is a double-edge sword. We have to learn how to use only the edge facing the enemy, the uncontrolled source.

◆ You do not drive in a foreign country without a map; why should you explore a previously operated abdomen without consulting the operative note?

◆ When the wound scar looks mature so are the adhesions inside; supple and bloodless.

◆ It is painful to re-operate on your own complications; it is fun to do on complications of another surgeon.

◆ He who operates and runs away, may get to re-operate on the same patient another day.

Chapter 75

Reputation

1   A slight touch of the cynic in manner and habits, gives the physician, to the common eye, an air of authority, which greatly tends to enlarge his reputation.
Walter Scott, 1771-1832

2   Any surgeon, who looks for repute to the general public, rather than to his own professional brothers, has the spirit of the quack.
J Chalmers Da Costa, 1863-1933

3   The reputation of a surgeon, in the final analysis, must rest upon: originality; teaching by word of mouth; teaching by the printed word; and operative skill.
William J Mayo, 1861-1939

4   A true surgeon is never fearless. He fears for his patients, he fears for his shortcomings, his own mistakes, but he never fears for himself or his professional reputation.
Samuel J Mixter, 1880-1958

Look wise, say nothing, and grunt. Speech was given to conceal thought.

William Osler, 1849-1919

Too good to be true, or too true to be good.

William Heneage Ogilvie, 1887-1971

Chapter 76

Research

1   I think your solution is just; but why think? Why not try the experiment?
John Hunter, 1728-1793

2   In the collection of evidence upon any medical subject, there are but three sources from which we can hope to obtain it: from observation of the living subject; from examination of the dead; and from experiment upon living animals.
Astley Paston Cooper, 1768-1841

3   He who combines the knowledge of physiology and surgery, in addition to the artistic side of his subject, reaches the highest ideal in medicine.
Theodor Billroth, 1829-1894

4   He who cannot quote his therapeutic experiences in numbers is a charlatan; be truthful for clarity's sake, do not hesitate to admit failures, as they must show the mode and places of improvement.
Theodor Billroth, 1829-1894

5   Now and then a very learned article or lecture, like the talk of the mass mentioned in Wolfville, increases the sum total of human ignorance.

J Chalmers Da Costa, 1863-1933

6   It is given to a few of us to be Columbuses of great continents of surgery - given to but few to discover such a principle as antisepsis as did Lord Lister - but all of us have at times our small triumphs, all of us are workers in the cause and all of us add something to knowledge.

J Chalmers Da Costa, 1863-1933

7   Some men are most ingenious in finding forgotten ideas and putting them forth as new and original. This process is, in reality, getting scientific eggs from cold storage and selling them as newly laid.

J Chalmers Da Costa, 1863-1933

8   A discovery is rarely, if ever, a sudden achievement, nor is it the work of one man; a long series of observations, each in turn received in doubt and discussed in hostility, are familiarized by time, and lead at last to the gradual disclosure of truth.

Berkeley Moynihan, 1865-1936

9   Only by passing through the fire of experiment will medicine as a whole become what it should be, namely, a conscious and, hence, always purposefully acting science.

Ivan Pavlov, 1849-1936

10 The scientist is not content to stop at the obvious.

Charles H Mayo, 1865-1939

11 Scientific truth, which I formerly thought of as fixed, as though it could be weighted and measured, is changeable. Add a fact, change the outlook, and you have a new truth.

William J Mayo, 1861-1939

12 The first attribute of a surgeon is an insatiable curiosity.

Russell John Howard, 1875-1942

13   One can accept a purely practical or a purely theoretical life ... one may practice the art upon suffering humanity or prosecute the science, upon which practice rests, in the absolute solitude of the laboratory. One life is filled with multivarious humanity, with the closest association with men; the other may be as isolated as that of religious hermits who live in mountain caves and reckon their devotion according to their isolation.

Elliot Carr Cutler, 1888-1947

14   An active clinical surgical position with its responsibilities for human life does not permit serious investigative work to be conducted at the same time.

Elliot Carr Cutler, 1888-1947

15   Medical scientists are nice people, but you should not let them treat you.

August Bier, 1861-1949

16   It is too bad that we cannot cut the patient in half in order to compare two regimens of treatment.

Béla Schick, 1877-1967

17   The surgeon's ideas, even if abstract, must be put into practice before they can be judged. The man who puts his thoughts into action will always excite opposition, for the mind is more conscious of the effect of deeds than words.

William E Tanner, 1889-?

18   The statement "all patients operated upon in this manner survived" probably means that any patient who died must *ipso facto* not have been operated upon "in this manner" and may therefore be excluded from the series.

Mark M Ravitch, 1910-1989

19   If you are going to peddle bovine shit, at least you should package it well.

Robert M Zollinger, 1903-1992

20   The surgical investigator must be a bridge tender, channeling knowledge from biologic science to the patient's bedside and back again. He traces his origin from both ends of the bridge. He is thus a bastard, and is called this by everybody. Those at one end of the bridge say that he is not a very good scientist, and those at the other end say he does not spend enough time in the operating room.

Francis D Moore, 1913-2001

21   Research of both kinds can be sloppy, dishonest, self-serving, or fraudulent.

Francis D Moore, 1913-2001

22   A statistical analysis, properly conducted, is a delicate dissection of uncertainties, a surgery of suppositions.

MJ Moroney

23   It is easier to obtain grants for imaginary things than real problems. The former feeds thoughts on success while the reality is known and unsolvable.

PO Nyström

24   One cannot be brief about a subject unless one knows it well.

Mary Evans

25   Surgeons were slow to embrace the new technique, possibly because of their self-perceived image of infallibility. One of the first honest doubters who saw the merits of the random control trial in surgical research was a colorectal surgeon, John Goligher. Thirty years ago he appreciated the three fundamental rules: that a trial must be prospective with contemporary controls randomized by a method that cannot be influenced by the investigator, that it must have a single objective clearly stated, and that it must have a potential for altering clinical practice.

Mary Evans

26   Definition of a double blind trial: two orthopaedic surgeons trying to read an ECG (EKG for our American colleagues).

Nick J Taffinder

27   Does absence of proof of efficacy provide proof of the absence of efficacy?

John Marshall

28 A single significant discovery during a lifetime of research means success.

Frank Mann

29 The purpose of a retrospective study is to kick us in the head, to challenge an assumption and to stimulate the design of a study that will generate class one data.

Michael McGonigal

30 The size of a clinic, an institute, the number of grants - obtained by all kinds of tricks - have little to do with creativity. Often activism and gigantism are mistaken for research.

Hans Troidl

31 Conceptually, the surgeon and bench scientist differ in three ways. 1. The scientist knows that he does not know, whereas the clinical surgeon treating patients is expected to know. 2. The scientist can wait for all the data to become available, whereas the surgeon must make a decision based on available data. 3. The scientist deals with mass data, whereas the surgeon deals with an individual patient.

Joseph E Murray

32 Nothing spoils good results as much as follow-up.

B Ramana

33 Do not let the data get in the way of your opinions.

Philip Barie

34 Trying to compare your numbers with the Mayo Clinic is as farting against the hurricane.

35 The more the noise, the less the fact.

36 If we don't describe it first, our first reaction is always negative.

37   The pleural of ANECDOTE is not DATA.

38   Surgical advance is something, which, if tested in a rat will produce a publication. It is a surgical innovation when the rat survives.

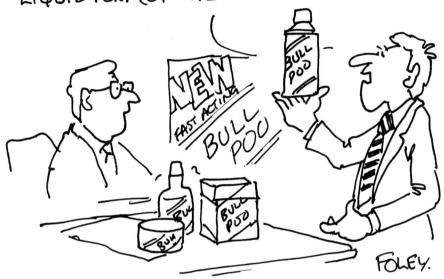

...AND THIS IS THE PACK DESIGN FOR THE LIQUID FORM OF THE PRODUCT.

If you are going to peddle bovine shit, at least you should package it well.

From the editor

◆ Suspect the retrospective study, which reports a zero mortality rate in X number of octogenarians: it only means the first and last mortalities were not included.

◆ As surgical procedures are evolving so rapidly there is a very narrow interval between when the surgical technology is too immature to test in randomized studies and when it is so well entrenched that surgeons are reluctant to randomize their patients.

Believe nobody -

question

everything.

Chapter 77

Responsibility

1 Drinking, whoring, and gambling should not be indulged in by the surgeon, for because of them he may well forget or omit something today concerning the patient which cannot be corrected tomorrow.
Wilhelm Fabry von Hilden, 1560-1624

2 One man alone and only one should be in charge of a case ... two men in charge is a surgical duet and like a musical duet is an arrangement by which each one may lay blame on the other.
J Chalmers Da Costa, 1863-1933

3 The surgeon may in some degree share his responsibilities with others, but the chief responsibility must always lie with him. And being his must be exercised not only during the operation but also before, perhaps long before, and also after, perhaps long after, the operation is performed.
Berkeley Moynihan, 1865-1936

4   A major difference between responsibility of pilot and surgeon is that the former shares directly in the consequences of his error or neglect, while the latter does not.

John S Lockwood, 1907-1950

5   Other people's life is a serious responsibility; one's own frequently not. Don't get this mixed up.

Charles FM Saint, 1886-1973

6   The surgeon, like the captain of the ship or a pilot of an aircraft, is responsible for everything that happened. His word is the only one that cannot be gainsaid.

Francis D Moore, 1913-2001

7   And he is alone. No matter how many others crowd about the mouth of the wound, no matter their admiration and encouragement, it is he that rappels this crevasse, dangles in this dreadful place, and he is afraid - for he knows well the worth of this belly, that it is priceless and irreplaceable.

Richard Selzer

8   Believe nobody - question everything.

9   Everybody's business is nobody's business.

10   Surgery is done by a committee of one.

Ventilate, perfuse,

and piss is all that

it is about.

Matt Oliver

Chapter 78

SICU

1   In acute diseases, coldness of the extremities is bad.

Hippocrates, 460-377 BC

2   The major cause of shock is decreased circulatory volume. Replace body fluids by the best means at hand.

Alfred Blalock, 1899-1964

3   Ventilate, perfuse, and piss is all that it is about.

Matt Oliver

4   Lack of urine output in the acutely hypovolemic patient is renal success, not renal failure.

Ronald V Maier

5   Anytime you are making love you have - per definition - SIRS

Arthur E Baue

6   Our ingenuity in developing terminology exceeds our abilities to take care of these patients once they have developed the syndrome of MOF. The solution to MOF or MODS or SIRS is prevention.

Arthur E Baue

7   Hospital-acquired generalized interstitial edema (HAGIE) as an acceptable, even necessary, consequence of modern resuscitation and parenteral fluid therapy needs to be recognized for what it is: the unwelcome consequence of uncontrolled resuscitation.

William Lyons

8   Chances of survival drops as the BUN exceeds the body weight.

Stephen J Prevoznik

9   The more the ECG resembles the EEG, the sicker the heart.

Stephen J Prevoznik

10   It is much easier to add drugs than to subtract them.

Stephen J Prevoznik

11   Surgeons are intensivists who operate or complete their training.

12   On fancy monitoring: we do not need a compass to find our way home.

13   On resuscitation: if you can't keep the patients alive when they are alive you can't keep them alive when they are dead.

14   The dumbest kidney is smarter than the smartest doctor.

15   Concerning the oxygen dissociation curve: anything, which shifts the curve to the right, is right.

16   A surgical airway is better than an arrested patient with a nice-looking neck. Halitosis is better than no breath at all.

17   Hypoxia not only stops the motor, it wrecks the engine.

From the editor

◆ The phenomenon of the surgical ostrich treating his patients for pneumonia while they are slowly sinking into multiple organ failure from poorly controlled surgical infection, still provides us a constant source of SICU experience.

◆ In sick surgical patients, unlike the medical ones, optimization means volume and more volume; a lot of fluids.

Chapter 79

Specialist

1   The definition of a specialist as one who "knows more and more about less and less" is good and true. Its truth makes essential that the specialist, to do efficient work, must have some association with others who, taken together, represent the whole of which the specialty is only a part.
Charles H and Charles W Mayo, 1865-1939

2   To my sons: whatever specialty they follow, may they never forget to be doctors.
Harry E Mock, 1880-?

3   Specialization is of greatest value to surgery, not because each branch studies some small subject with greater intensity, but because each brings a fresh outlook, a new school of surgical thought, which can be supplied with benefit to the rest of the art.
William Heneage Ogilvie, 1887-1971

Everybody is against specialization except the patient.

Francis D Moore,

1913-2001

4   The most important contribution a specialist can make is to say the patient's disease is not in his domain.

Mark M Ravitch, 1910-1989

5   Everybody is against specialization except the patient.

Francis D Moore, 1913-2001

6   Domination by one specialty is not healthy for either public service or the balance of teaching. Domination becomes damnation.

Francis D Moore, 1913-2001

7   All you have to do to be a neurosurgeon is know that the brain forks and that air rises.

Saul Rosen

Chapter 80

Speed

Fast surgeons do not hurry, they save time by not wasting motions.

1   The physician can do all he has to do with speed and precision, but he must never appear to be in a hurry, and never absent-minded.

Theodor Billroth, 1829-1894

2   Surgeons who take unnecessary risks and operate by the clock are exciting from the onlooker's standpoint, but they are not necessarily those in whose hands you would by preference choose to place yourself.

Theodor Kocher, 1841-1917

3   There is no need ... to be rash or daring, but let them be foresighted, gentle and circumspect, in order that with the greatest deliberateness and gentleness they may operate under all circumstances with what gentleness they can.

William Stewart Halsted, 1852-1922

4   The worship of efficiency is the destruction of individualism ... to destroy individualism is in the long run to destroy civilization. A nation devoted purely to efficiency is a nation of brutes bent on savagery.

J Chalmers Da Costa, 1863-1933

5   Observers no longer expect to be thrilled in an operating room; the spectacular public performances of the past, no longer condoned, are replaced by the quiet, rather tedious procedures, which few beyond the operator, his assistants, and the immediate bystander can profitably see. The patient on the table, like the passenger in a car, runs greater risks if he has a loquacious driver, or one who takes close corners, exceeds the speed limit, or rides to admiration.

Harvey Williams Cushing, 1869-1939

6   Speed in operating should be the achievement, not the aim, of every surgeon.

Russell John Howard, 1875-1942

7   Waste of time must be avoided, but very often, when a difficulty is encountered, the time lost by a pause to appraise the situation is compensated by a job better done afterwards.

William Heneage Ogilvie, 1887-1971

8   Every surgeon has his own normal speed, and to hurry is likely to produce deterioration in the quality of his work.

Charles FM Saint, 1886-1973

9   In the long pace of days and weeks and the long years of human life with remembrance of things past and apprehension of things to come, it is hard to remember that in preserving human life there are occasions when seconds count, minutes are too long.

Francis D Moore, 1913-2001

10   When I am carrying out a big, unusual, or difficult operation, I never plan anything later that day.

Francis D Moore, 1913-2001

11   Operate in haste - repent in leisure.

Phil Caropreso

12   Speed is achieved by precision not precipitation.

Nita Costescu

13   To get good and fast, first you must get good; afterward you will get fast. If you get good, you will never really need to get fast, but if you are fast and not really good, it's really bad. Nuff said?

Tom Horan

14   Any operation takes longer than the surgeon says it will.

Clifton K Meador

15   *Despacio voy, porque de prisa estoy.* Slowly I go because I am in a hurry.

Eric Olivero

16   Hurry we have to finish the operation before he dies.

17   When in a hurry - slow down.

18   Speed is nothing but economy of movements.

19   Fast surgeons do not hurry, they save time by not wasting motions.

From the editor

◆   As the Italians say: "*chi va piano va lontano*" - the one who walks slowly walks far.

In the VA

Hospital:

whatever you

need, you won't

get. Whatever

you'll get is worth

shit.

From the movie -

Article 99

Chapter 81

Standard of care

1   It is rather dangerous for a surgeon to operate differently than is the custom of the other surgeons ... we have suffered the disdain of shameful words on the part of laymen and of our colleagues, the surgeons; and even threats and dangers.
    Henri de Mondeville, 1260-1320

2   Surgical procedure cannot be standardized, applied at random and the result invariably predicted. To remove a gallbladder or drain a pelvic abscess is not the same operation in any two individuals, for no two patients are alike, physically, psychologically or surgically.
    Max Thorek, 1880-1960

3   There can be no malpractice without established practice; a physician cannot be convicted of deviating from accepted standards if no accepted standards exist.
    James C Mohr

Chapter 82

Statistics

1   Statistics are like women; mirrors of purest virtue and truth, or like whores, to use as one pleases.
Theodor Billroth, 1829-1894

2   Statistics, which, if properly collected and set forth, are immensely valuable, are often but the dull man's delight. The little items, "excluded cases" and "moribund cases" are common in statistical tables, and like charity, they cover a multitude of sins.
J Chalmers Da Costa, 1863-1933

3   Some purveyors of statistics are fine imaginative writers and should be war correspondents.
J Chalmers Da Costa, 1863-1933

4   Statistics don't lie, but the men who make them sometimes do.
J Chalmers Da Costa, 1863-1933

The fact that a stone, thrown out of the window, rises instead of falls is not statistically significant, but it is a powerful observation.

Nicola Basso

5   Statistics will prove anything, even the truth.

Berkeley Moynihan, 1865-1936

6   Even a sensible person promptly associates the term "statistics" with the thought: "this is a bunch of lies".

August Bier, 1861-1949

7   Personal statistics are at the bottom of all unsound teaching; they are either too good to be true or too true to be good.

William Heneage Ogilvie, 1887-1971

8   The only figures which I find statistically significant are those recorded anonymously and analyzed impartially by someone with no personal interest in the verdict.

William Heneage Ogilvie, 1887-1971

9   If your first essay at an operation results in fatality it will take a long time to get good statistics.

Mark M Ravitch, 1910-1989

10   The fact that a stone, thrown out of the window, rises instead of falls is not statistically significant, but it is a powerful observation.

Nicola Basso

11   Medical statistics are like a bikini. What they reveal is interesting but what they conceal is vital.

12   You don't need to run Chi Square on common sense.

13   Medical statistics are a special branch of alchemy, carefully crafted to turn bullshit to airline tickets.

14   If you torture the data long enough, you can make it say anything.

Chapter 83

Stomach, Duodenum & Esophagus

1 Etiology of an ulcer: either a naughty or irregular diet or the ill disposition of entrails.
Ambroise Paré, 1510-1590

2 Cancerous disorganization of the stomach, in some instances, gives no indication of its existence, sufficiently distinct to render its detection possible, during life, even by the most compelling and careful observers.
Elisha Bartlett, 1804-1855

3 The brain secretes thought as the stomach secretes gastric juice, the liver bile, and the kidneys urine.
Karl Vogt, 1817-1895

4 Every doctor, faced with a perforated ulcer of the stomach or intestine, must consider opening the abdomen, sewing up the hole, and averting a possible or actual inflammation by careful cleansing of the abdominal cavity.
Johan Mikulicz-Radecki, 1850-1905

In the era of Helicobacter pylori doing a gastrectomy for peptic ulcer is like doing a lobectomy for pneumonia.

Asher Hirshberg

5   No acid, no ulcer.

K Schwartz, ~1910

6   I do not know any operation in surgery which gives better results, which gives more complete satisfaction, both to the patient and his surgeon, than gastroenterostomy for chronic ulcer of the stomach.

Berkeley Moynihan, 1865-1936

7   If anyone should consider removing half of my good stomach to cure a small ulcer in my duodenum, I would run faster than he.

Charles H Mayo, 1865-1939

8   We have no responsibility to such patients but to save their lives. Any procedure, which aims to do more than this, can quite significantly be considered meddlesome surgery. We have no responsibility during the surgery to carry out any procedure to cure the patient of his original duodenal ulcer.

Roscoe R Graham, 1890-1948

9   In ten-fifteen years when the final bad results of vagotomy will have been evaluated, the operation will be in the same category as gastroenterostomy.

Alton J Oschner, 1896-1981

10   About gastrectomy for duodenal ulcer: in this operation ... a segment of an essentially normal stomach is removed to treat the disease next door in the duodenum. It is like taking out the engine to decrease noise in the gear box.

Francis D Moore, 1913-2001

11   Separate a man's desire for food from his ability to ingest it and you have dysphasia. Interrupt the pathway from the mouth to belly and you have an alarming symptom for which a patient usually seeks advice without delay.

PB Nelson

12 Osler referred to duodenal ulcer as "the wound stripe of civilization". Perhaps we are becoming less civilised.

Edward R Woodward

13 In the era of *Helicobacter pylori* doing a gastrectomy for peptic ulcer is like doing a lobectomy for pneumonia.

Asher Hirshberg

14 It is an interesting fact that practically every operative procedure which has been advocated as a method of therapy for bleeding esophageal varices has a small percentage of salvaged cases.

R Cohn

15 Perforated ulcer: there is a hole in my bucket ... how should I mend it? Just patch it!

A folk song

From the editor

◆ When the blood is fresh and pink and the patient is old, it is time to be active and bold. When the patient is young and the blood is dark and old, you can relax and put your knife on hold.

◆ Doing a gastrectomy for an ulcer is to produce another disease.

◆ Too much or too little of anything is not good, including wine, other things and perhaps acid.

As a surgeon one

is an optimist -

otherwise one

would not be a

surgeon.

Karl H Bauer,

1890-1978

Chapter 84

Surgeons

1 Should be cleanly in his habits and well shaved, and should not allow his nails to grow. He should wear white garments ... and walk about with a mild and benignant look as a friend of all well beings.
Sushruta, <8th century, BC

2 The surgeon should have a perceptive eye, ideas that are always lucid, of the nature that will enable him always to act with promptness and assurance.
Jean Yperman, 1260-1310

3 The conditions necessary for the surgeon are four: first, he should be learned; second, he should be expert; third, he must be ingenious, and fourth, he should learn to adapt himself.
Guy de Chauliac, 1300-1368

4 You should also wear good clothes but you should not be vain so that the patients trust you the more and derive hope from you, for hope is what the patients desire.
Hieronymus Brunschwig, 1450-1512

5   A pitiful surgeon makes a dangerous sore.

John Marston, 1575-1634

6   It is the surgeon's duty to tranquillize the temper, to beget cheerfulness, and to impact confidence of recovery.

Astley Paston Cooper 1768-1841

7   Surgeons ... spend raptures upon perfect specimens of indurated veins, distorted joints, or beautiful new cases of curved spine.

Elizabeth B Browning, 1806-1861

8   The drunkard surgeon is the licensed assassin.

Frank Hastings Hamilton, 1813-1886

9   A person may have learned a very great deal and still be an exceedingly unskilful physician, who awakens little confidence in his power.

Theodor Billroth, 1829-1894

10 A surgeon is judged by three A's: ability, availability and affability.

Paul Reznikoff, ~1896

11 Thus love, joy, ardor, courage, hate, fear, rage, passion, all seek expression which, unless directed by reason, may become a danger; love degenerating into passion, joy into orgy, ardor into impatience, and courage into recklessness.

Victor Horsley, 1857-1916

12 The ideal surgeon has not as yet been born ... he would have wisdom as well as knowledge - tact as well as skill - confident hope as well as cautious doubt. His hand, like that of Joseph Pancoast, would be as light as floating perfume - his eye as quick as light beam - his heart as broad as humanity - his soul as sweet as the waters of Lebanon.

J Chalmers Da Costa, 1863-1933

13 Fashionable surgeons are seldom great surgeons.

J Chalmers Da Costa, 1863-1933

14   Our most splendid triumphs, our worst mistakes, and our saddest failures come from the radical mind ... he has an utter contempt for authority ... he is never moderate, in fact, he scorns moderation ... he is invariably convinced that he is always right ... his knife may cut for good or ill. He obtains wonderful successes and makes dreadful mistakes. He is often a copious and hasty writer ... the best type of radical makes the real progress...

J Chalmers Da Costa, 1863-1933

15   The conservative is often a most valuable factor in surgery. He is a brake on the wheel and often stops the dashing automobile of progress when on a joy ride from upsetting in the ditch of folly ... he studies the past and reveres it ... he attaches an exaggerated importance to books, and minimises the value of new methods of communicating ideas. He has a great respect for authorities ... he is prone to write pondering treatises, each of which has a name so complicated that it sounds like a sobriety test ... he agrees with Solomon that there is no new thing.

J Chalmers Da Costa, 1863-1933

16   A vain surgeon is like a milking stool, of no use except when sat upon.

J Chalmers Da Costa, 1863-1933

17   The vain man in surgery is a deadly peril. He mistakes his own half-formed opinions for oracles speaking within him.

J Chalmers Da Costa, 1863-1933

18   Why do people become surgeons? Very few because of natural inclination, though some do. Most men have become surgeons because of a developed liking for it, because of some particular opportunity of some chance which stirred the idea. Often a son will adopt a father's speciality, as did the younger Gross, the younger Pancoast, and the younger Kocher.

J Chalmers Da Costa, 1863-1933

19   A man who doesn't worry at all doesn't care a whole lot. I should not want a man who did not care a whole lot operating on me or mine.

J Chalmers Da Costa, 1863-1933

20   Sometimes cowardice, sometimes laziness, sometimes selfishness saves a man from being called irritable, combative, and cantankerous. What a man doesn't do is not always a sign of what he is and isn't. We must know why he doesn't do it in order to reach a conclusion.

J Chalmers Da Costa, 1863-1933

21   I think all of us who have worked years in the profession understand that many very skillful operators are not good surgeons.

William J Mayo, 1861-1939

22   The surgeon is often intolerant and the internist self sufficient.

William J Mayo, 1861-1939

23   Medicine is about as big or as little in any community, large or small, as the physicians make it.

Charles H Mayo, 1865-1939

24   It is a good thing for a surgeon to have prematurely gray hair and itchy piles. The first makes him appear to know more than he does and the second gives him an expression of concern which the patient interprets as being on his behalf.

A Benson Cannon, 1889-1950

25   He was in bed before eleven-thirty; he never took more than one drink a day; and he never read anything or said anything which would not contribute to his progress as a Brilliant Young Surgeon.

Sinclair Lewis, 1885-1951

26   When I take up assassinations, I shall start with the surgeons in this city and work up to the gutter.

Dylan Thomas, 1914-1953

27   I prefer to be called a fool for asking the question rather than remain in ignorance.

John Homans, 1877-1954

28 The master surgeon must be a man of mind, a man of thought, a man who knows his province, the human body, as a whole and not only one of its parts.

Rudolph Matas, 1860-1957

29 He presents to me ... as a great surgeon before the days of anaesthetics, versed in every detail of such science as was known to him: sure of himself, steady of poise, knife in hand, intent upon the operation; entirely removed in his professional capacity from the agony of the patient, the anguish of relations, or the doctrines of rival schools, the devices of quacks, or the first-fruits of new learning.

Winston S Churchill, 1874-1965

30 I can practise in an honorary fashion the arts of surgery and medicine. Being temperamentally inclined to precision and a sharp edge, it might be thought that I should choose the surgeon's role.

Winston S Churchill, 1874-1965

31 A surgeon who is his own physician, though he often has a fool for a colleague, has the happiness of working in an atmosphere of mutual confidence and admiration.

William Heneage Ogilvie, 1887-1971

32 A bad surgeon is one who has inherited the trends but not the traditions of a great master, who has his mannerisms without his manners. He looks at disease through an endoscope. He speaks of cases not patients. He has no culture, no knowledge of the basic sciences, and therefore no breadth of vision. He knows all about operating except when to refrain.

William Heneage Ogilvie, 1887-1971

33 Surgeons are a little too apt to treat their art as an entrancing hobby, rather than an instrument capable of doing great good and unspeakable harm.

William Heneage Ogilvie, 1887-1971

34 The good surgeon is orthodox in his teaching and his public utterance; heterodox in his innermost conscience.

William Heneage Ogilvie, 1887-1971

35   The great surgeon is humble by nature, because the things he has done count for him as very little in comparison with the great mass of the things that yet remain to be done. He is slow to criticize others, yet tolerant of those who criticize him.

William Heneage Ogilvie, 1887-1971

36   You can't always be clever, but you can always be kind.

Charles Wilson Moran, 1882-1977

37   As a surgeon one is an optimist - otherwise one would not be a surgeon.

Karl H Bauer, 1890-1978

38   There are two groups of surgeons: those who see what they believe and those who believe what they see.

Owen H Wangensteen, 1898-1981

39   He did not have the extrovert character which is so often the mark of the successful surgeon.

Geoffrey Keynes, 1887-1982

40   Every surgeon is liable to have a dose of whatever by which he chiefly lives.

Geoffrey Keynes, 1887-1982

41   Beware the surgeon who is great at getting out of trouble.

Mark M Ravitch, 1910-1989

42   The expert surgeon is smarter than the algorithm.

Charles M Abernathy, 1941-1994

43   For the body hemostasis. For the mind, equanimity.

Francis D Moore, 1913-2001

44   I am an armchair surgeon, now retired from sheer boredom.

Ravindra Padmanabhan, 1950-2001

45   They found themselves classier tailors, the kind used by surgeons, professional athletes, and racketeers.

Saul Bellow

46   The specimens he removed were always heavier than the part of the patient he left behind.

Jim Howell

47   Call me when you run out of blood and morphine.

Ario Hermreck

48   No more *mea culpa*. *Mea culpa* belongs to a Latin mass.

Creighton Hardin

49   Don't go to a surgeon whose office plants have died.

Joseph Alberton

50   Talking of surgeons - how do you tell the difference between God and a surgeon? God knows He's not a surgeon!

Iain Thirsk

51   I still deeply feel that good surgeons are the last bastion of good medicine.

Mark Rogers

52   Surgeons are the fighter pilots of the medical profession.

Howard McCollister

53   He is like the surgeon who has grown tired of blood. He is content that others should operate.

John Le Carre

54   First, the abiding fear that someone will waste our time, because we must always appear to be busy and on the run; second, we may be wrong - but we are never in doubt.

Judah Folkman

55   The modern surgeon will never revert to the technical brute who was regarded as the mechanical arm of the medical profession. The "mechanical brute", however, must persist if the surgeon is to maintain an appropriate role.

Seymour I Schwartz

56   Nobody has come up with a good way of assessing surgeons, not for their competence (that's fairly easy), but for their performance. It is only the anesthesiologist who can offer an opinion about who is the gentle surgeon and who the butcher. Or is the answer, in the words of my friend Hiram C Polk, Jr. that surgeons who have extremely low rates of surgical site infection suffer from "selective forgetfulness"?

Allan Pollock

57   For a surgeon: modesty - the shortest way to obscurity.

Youry Vladimirovitch Plotnicov

58   It is not the surgeon who does not drink pure spirit, does not sleep with the scrub nurse and does not urinate in a washstand.

Youry Vladimirovitch Plotnicov

59   Every hospital seems to have an almost invariant cast of surgical characters: the Prima Donna, the Old-Time Surgeon, The Sleazy Surgeon, the Buffoon, the Compassionate Young Surgeon, the Exemplary Surgeon.

Joan Cassell

60   A surgeon requires immediate, rapid, and positive feedback; the intellectual interest of the problem, in and of itself, is rarely enough. We might speculate that the kind of person who becomes a doctor is someone who likes to be admired, while the kind of person who becomes a surgeon is someone who needs to be admired. Performing a miracle may be as essential to the self-image of the surgeon as to the well-being of the patient.

Joan Cassell

61   A surgeon is a physician who can't wait to get into the operating room and, once there, can't wait to get out.

Jonathan R Hiatt

62   The egotistical surgeon is like a monkey; the higher he climbs the more you see of his less attractive features.

63   The best surgeon is he that has been well hacked himself.

64   Surgeons are internists who operate.

65   If a surgeon were asked to name the three greatest surgeons, he would be hard-pressed to name the other two.

66   A very bold surgeon is one who does not realize that it is the patient who takes all the risks.

67   Impatient surgeons lose their patients.

68   If you see two surgeons laughing, someone is in trouble.

69   Clinical ego is the patient's enemy ... know when to back off and when to call for help.

70   Beware of colleagues with no sense of humor; they are never very bright and will blame you for their error.

71   You are never a prophet in your own hometown.

72   There is no better surgeon than one with many scars.

73   A touch of paranoia is healthy but not everyone wants to kill your patient.

74   Two thirds of surgery is competence, a third confidence.

75   You can take your work seriously but take yourself less so.

76   It is easy for a surgeon to grow cocky but hard to stay long this way.

77   Surgeons and soldiers see each other in their underwear, thus they differ from internists.

78   The bigger they are, the harder they fall.

79   A big surgeon; a big cemetery.

80   Surgery is a contact sport.

81   Operating is a highly addicting habit.

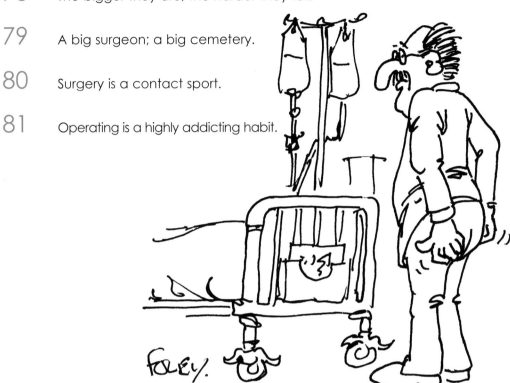

It is a good thing for a surgeon to have prematurely gray hair and itchy piles.....

From the editor

◆   Selecting a surgeon is like choosing a car: any car would bring you to your destination but in the event of an accident a Volvo or a Mercedes would increase your chances of survival.

◆   Physicians carry a stethoscope around their neck, surgeons not. Why? Surgeons do not need another long and heavy object to fortify their ego; they possess one already.

In surgery like in sex: don't complain about too much surgery because there will be times when you don't get enough.

Chapter 85

Surgery & Love

1   Surgeons and anatomists see no beautiful women in their lives, but only a ghastly stack of bones with Latin names to them, and a network of nerves and muscles and tissues inflamed by disease.
Mark Twain, 1835-1910

2   By the time a man really attains success in surgery, he is on the heights of middle age, and, like a woman in a bathing dress - he wants but little here below, nor wants that little long.
J Chalmers Da Costa, 1863-1933

3   Just as there are no great one-handed lovers, there are no great one-handed surgeons.
Howard McCollister

4   In surgery, as in love, never say never, never say always.
Jorge Bezama

5   The scrub nurse is a second wife of the surgeon.
Viatcheslav ("Slava") Ryndine

6   In surgery as in love, too much concentration on technique can often lead to impotence.

7   Surgery like lovemaking must be done gently and with adequate exposure.

8   In surgery like in sex: don't complain about too much surgery because there will be times when you don't get enough.

9   Working in a dark hole has its advantages but not in the operating room.

10   Not having the right instrument at the right time is like not having a condom; no point looking for it if you don't have it because by the time you find it you won't need it.

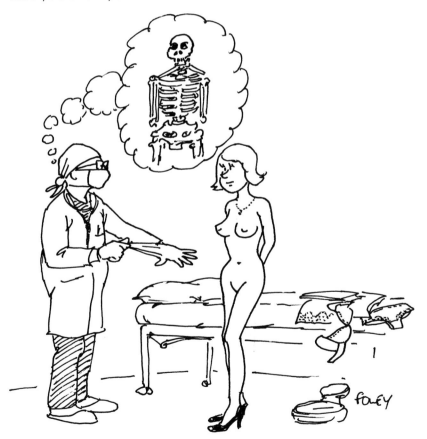

Surgeons and anatomists see no beautiful women in their lives, but only a ghastly stack of bones.....

Recurrent nerve

at thyroidectomy:

not seen, not

caught.

Bernard Cristalli

Chapter 86

Thyroid

1   Everyday, morning and evening the setons are drawn towards the outside until finally the flesh is cut through. When this is done if any part of the goiter remains, powder it.

Roland of Parma, ~1170

2   I have lately seen three cases of violent and long continued palpitations in females, in each of which the same peculiarity presented itself, viz: enlargement of the thyroid gland ... it was observed that the eyes assumed a singular appearance, for the eyeballs were apparently enlarged, so that when she slept or tried to shut her eyes, the lids were incapable of closing.

Robert J Graves, 1796-1853

3   No sensible man will, on slight consideration, attempt to extirpate a goitrous thyroid gland. If a surgeon should be so adventurous or foolhardy as to undertake the enterprise, I shall not envy him his feelings while engaged in the performance of it, or after he has completed it, should he be so fortunate as to do this. Every step he takes will be environed with difficulty, every stroke of his knife will be followed by a torrent of blood and lucky will it be for him if his victim lives long enough to enable him to finish his horrid butchery.

Samuel Gross, 1805-1884

4   The extirpation of the thyroid gland for goiter typifies, perhaps better than any operation, the supreme triumph of the surgeon's art. A feat which today can be accomplished by any really competent operator without danger of mishap and which was conceived more than 1000 years ago.

William Stewart Halsted, 1852-1922

5   Recurrent nerve at thyroidectomy: not seen, not caught.

Bernard Cristalli

In this operation,

bleeding cannot cause

any embarrassment,

because in cutting the

skin, there is very,

very little blood, and

in cutting the trachea,

none whatsoever

comes forth.

**Hieronymus
Fabricius ab Aquapendente,
1533-1620**

Chapter 87

Tracheostomy

1   We slit ... open a part of the arteria aspera (trachea) below the top of the windpipe, about the third or fourth ring. For this is a convenient situation, as being free of flesh, and because the vessels are placed at a distance from the part which is divided .... we judge that the windpipe has been opened from the air rushing through it with a whizzing noise, and from the voice being lost.

Paul of Aegina, 625-690

2   Many physicians are averse to this operation, either estimating it dangerous, deadly, or inhumane. But those gentlemen are greatly mistaken: for the small wound made in the trachea by this operation, is so far from killing.

Lorenz Heister, 1683-1758

Chapter 88

Trauma

Trauma is the motor end plate of violence.

Claude H Organ

1 An injury to the head is never so slight as to be despised, and never so severe as to be despaired of.
    Hippocrates, 460-377 BC

2 Physicians have to act not only in the cities, in the field, and in the desert places, but also at sea in ships, where such diseases sometimes suddenly break out.
    Paul of Aegina, 625-690

3 He should have a special love for the wounded persons as for his own body.
    Hans von Gersdorff, 1480-1540

4 It is absolutely necessary for a surgeon to search the wound himself, which were not drest by him at first, in order to discover their nature and know their extent.
    Augustine Belloste, 1645-1730

5   Wounds in the joints are always dangerous.

John Ranby, 1703-1773

6   A gunshot wound is often not completely understood at first, for it is at first, in many cases, impossible to know what parts are killed … till the deadened part has separated, which often makes it a much more complicated wound than at first was known or imagined.

John Hunter, 1728-1793

7   On fistula from an injured abdominal viscus: this new symptom, although in general very disagreeable, will not be dangerous, for all the danger is over before it can appear.

John Hunter, 1728-1793

8   We will always start with the most dangerously injured without regard to rank and distinction.

Jean Larrey, 1766-1842

9   That is the best country which has the fewest diseases, laws and crime.

Karl Marx, 1796-1877

10   Exploratory laparotomy offers, in our judgment, the quickest and the safest method of positive diagnosis. The emergency warrants a decisive step.

Albert Miles, ~1893

11   How varied was our experience of the battlefield and how fertile the blood of warriors in rearing good surgeons.

Thomas Clifford Allbutt, 1836-1925

12   Splint them where they lie.

Anthony A Bowlby, 1855-1929

13   Shock from severe wounds and hemorrhage always must take precedence of everything else.

William W Keen, 1837-1932

14   It seems that there will always be a surgery of war. This will contribute as much to progress as war itself.

Harvey Graham, ~1939

15   More limbs and lives are lost at the front from the improper use of the tourniquet than are saved by its proper use.

Douglas Jolly, ~1939

16   It is highly desirable that anyone engaged in war surgery should keep his ideas fluid and so be ready to abandon methods which prove unsatisfactory in favor of others which, at first, may appear revolutionary and even not free from inherent danger.

HH Sampson, ~1940

17   Doubt as to the condition of the wound should incline one to pessimism rather than to mistaken optimism.

William Heneage Ogilvie, 1887-1971

18   Simple closure of a wound of the colon, however small, is not warranted.

William Heneage Ogilvie, 1887-1971

19   A chain is only as strong as its weakest link ... the obvious weakest link in the severely wounded in this war (W.W.II) was the kidney.

Edward D Churchill, 1895-1972

20   During each latter war I watched surgeons committing the same errors I learned to avoid during 1941. Such a waste in young lives.

Karl Schein, 1911-1974

21   Death and taxes are the two most quoted inevitabilities of life; trauma qualifies as a legitimised third.

Alexander J Walt, 1923-1996

22   Surgery is a controlled trauma under anaesthesia.

Dag Sørlie

23   Even a dead patient's vital signs are stable.

William M Bowling

24   In any emergency setting, confusion is a function of the cube (N^3) of the number of people involved.

Clement A Hiebert

25   Failure to promptly recognize and treat simple life-threatening injuries is the tragedy of trauma, not the inability to handle the catastrophic or complicated injury.

F William Blaisdell

26   Trauma is the motor end plate of violence.

Claude H Organ

27   If the tattoo-teeth ratio is >1 the prognosis is favourable.

28   One set of vital signs isn't "hemodynamically stable".

29   The life you save may take your own.

Chapter 89

Truth

1   The principle, method and the goal of investigations is recognition of the truth, even though the truth may be in conflict with our social, ethical and public circumstances.
Theodor Billroth, 1829-1894

2   A doctor should always tell the truth; he should not hide it, for the patient is entitled to know the truth.
Johan Mikulicz-Radecki, 1850-1905

3   Next to the promulgation of the truth, the best thing I can conceive that a man can do is the public recantation of an error.
Joseph Lister, 1827-1912

4   Men tried to add to and adorn the truth, and convert simplicity into complexity and the clear into the opaque. Hence, the development of an enormous number of entirely unnecessary additions to the methods of surgery - additions so numerous and complicated that few know them all and none understood them all.
J Chalmers Da Costa, 1863-1933

A new truth does not triumph by convincing its opponents...but rather because they eventually die.

Max Planck, 1858-1947

5   A new truth does not triumph by convincing its opponents ... but rather because they eventually die.

Max Planck, 1858-1947

6   Where the truth lies? Not in numbers, for a small series carefully observed and recorded by a critical expert may mean more than several hundreds furnished by a team and analysed by slide rule. Not in the magic of a name, for truth may lie in the contribution of the small town practitioner, penned apologetically and hidden in the pages of a little read journal, rather than in the figures hammered out by platinum secretaries in the chromium laboratories of the million dollar professor.

William Heneage Ogilvie, 1887-1971

7   Should not established authorities ... accept the fact that many truths will be proved false, and aphorisms are better set in sand than in stone, and that the maverick of the present will contribute to the development of a new mean and new credo for the future.

Seymour I Schwarz

8   It's just easier to offer false hope than bitter truth.

Mark Pleatman

9   The ABCs of any M & M conference are: Accuse, Blame, Criticize, Defend (yourself), Evade truth.

From the editor ◆ Our sick patients are very complex. Events follow in a rush. But behind this complex chaos there is always an eternal truth that should be and can be disclosed and announced.

Chapter 90

Unnecessary

1   A possible apprehension now is that the surgeon be sometimes tempted to supplant instead of aiding nature.
Henry Maudsley, 1835-1918

2   The surgical cycle in women: appendix removed, right kidney hooked up, gallbladder taken out, gastroenterostomy, clean sweep of uterus and adnexa.
William Osler, 1849-1919

3   Martin would without fear have submitted ... for any operation of the head or neck, providing he was himself quite sure that the operation was necessary, but he was never able to rise to the clinic's faith that any portion of the body without which people could conceivably get along should certainly be removed at once.
Sinclair Lewis, 1885-1951

4   The so-called surgeon who practises primarily for the fee, who advises operation without adequate study, who removes a normal organ without indication, who makes an emergency out of almost every case, has no problems or morals.
Edwin P Lehman, 1888-1954

The surgical cycle in women: appendix removed, right kidney hooked up, gallbladder taken out, gastroenterostomy, clean sweep of uterus and adnexa.

William Osler,
1849-1919

5   The lowest mortality and fewest complications result from the removal of normal tissue.

Mark M Ravitch, 1910-1989

6   If your only tool is a hammer the whole world looks like a nail.

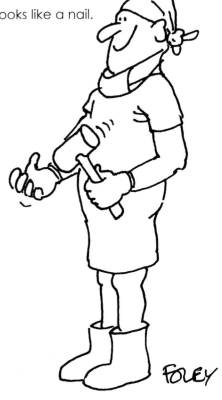

If your only tool is a hammer the whole world looks like a nail.

From the editor

◆   Real surgeons do only what is necessary; only jerks fortify their faltering egos with layers of unnecessary steps: another CT, another consultation, another blood test, another week of AB, another 20 liters of lavage, another 2 units of blood transfusion, another liter of bloodletting, another two drains.

Chapter 91

Vessels

1   There are two kinds of aneurysms. In the first the artery has undergone a local dilatation; in the second the artery has been ruptured. The aneurysms which are due to dilatation are longer than the others. The aneurysms by rupture are more rounded.
Antyllus, second century AD

2   To refuse to treat any aneurysm ... is unwise; but it is also dangerous to operate upon all of them.
Antyllus, second century AD

3   In the case of an (venous) ulcer, it is not expedient to stand; more especially if the ulcer is situated in the leg.
Celsus, 25BC-AD50

4   If the weapon had lodged in any of the larger vessels, such as the internal jugulars or carotids, and the large arteries in the armpits or groins. And if the extraction

Do not place your trust in the graft but also search carefully the host factors into which it is implanted. They may be decisive.

Henry Haimovici

threatens a great haemorrhage, they are first to be secured with ligatures on both sides, and then the extraction is to be made.

Paul of Aegina, 625-690

5   Veins which by the thickening of their tunicles in the old restrict the passage of blood, and by this lack of nourishment destroy their life without any fever, the old coming to fail little by little in slow death.

Leonardo da Vinci, 1452-1519

6   An aneurysm is the dilatation of an artery full of spirituous blood.

Jean Fernel, 1506-1558

7   The man is as old as his arteries.

Thomas Sydenham, 1624-1689

8   The vein will be dilated or become varicose, and it will have a pulsatile jarring on account of the stream from the artery. It will make a hissing noise, which will be found to correspond with the pulse ... it is like what is produced in the mouth by continuing the sound of the letter "R" in a whisper.

William Hunter, 1718-1783

9   Do not mistake the line of discoloration in gangrene for the line of demarcation. The former spreads, the latter rarely moves.

Augustus Charles Bernays, 1854-1907

10   Varicose veins are the results of an improper selection of grandparents.

William Osler, 1849-1919

11   A porter who had a huge aneurysm of the common iliac artery was admitted to Guy's. The next day the porter's aneurysm ruptured ... Astley Cooper saw the patient a little later ... and the man was slowly dying. He had a chance in a million of surviving, if the surgeon was courageous enough ... to operate on him would be near murder, yet not to operate would be to deny the man the last hope of even a few hours more of life. The surgeon turned to the

students who pressed about him: "gentlemen, this only hope of safety I am determined to give him". The operation took only a few minutes. The aorta was ligated just above the aneurysm. Three hours later the man was fairly well. The next morning he was sitting up in bed smiling ... in the afternoon, however, he died.

Harvey Graham, ~1939

12   Vascular surgery is peculiar because, above all, it is mainly surgery of ruins.

Cid dos Santos

13   You do not sleep too well the night before a bad AAA - you do not sleep well the night after a distal bypass.

Angus McIver

14   Do not place your trust in the graft but also search carefully the host factors into which it is implanted. They may be decisive.

Henry Haimovici

15   Some arteries are close and available, others hidden and protected. Some are soft, supple and forgiving; others hard, unyielding, and foreboding ... the aneurysm is a beast, large, looming, and threatening. It heaves with every heart beat, steam rising, paying no mind. Grasp it at the throat, open it quickly, exposing its innards, the debris of life. The carotid ... is graceful, quiet and restrained, full of mystery. Touch it gently.

Bruce J Brener

16   It always starts with a fem-pop; then it becomes a fem-chop.

Sai Sajja

17   Abdominal pain and hypotension equals a ruptured AAA, unless proven otherwise.

18   It is better to see the outside of the artery before you see the inside.

19   Arterial spasm is spelled clot.

20 The first and second rules of vascular surgery: proximal and distal control.

21 Use balloon embolectomy like the toilet paper: keep passing it until you don't get anymore.

22 You can't make a palpable pulse more palpable.

23 A macho surgeon: "the only blood vessel I can't Bovie is the aorta".

24 It is safer to leave an artery ungrafted than to endarterectomize it.

25 Atherosclerosis is like a cancer of the vessels.

26 In senile gangrene do not neglect the only drug of use - Opium; give it while you are awaiting the time to do an amputation high up.

From the editor

◆ In vascular surgery all you need to know is the site of the lesion, number of segments involved, the inflow, the runoff and the general status of the patient.

◆ A patient does not need a functioning graft to sit in a wheel chair or lie in a bed; a stump of amputation would do.

◆ When you ask a vascular surgeon to justify unnecessary surgery he'll cite from the following: we tried to save his leg, he had rest pain, his aneurysm was painful, she had TIAs, and always - the family wanted us to do whatever we could.

◆ A fresh wound of a failed bypass graft procedure is not a prerequisite to amputation.

◆ In ruptured AAAs the operation is commonly the beginning of the end with the end arriving post-operatively.

◆ Resuscitation in a ruptured AAA means an aortic clamp above the aneurysm.

Chapter 92

VIP

I hope my surgeon

is a republican.

Ronald Reagan

1 Operating on King George IV's infected sebaceous cyst of the scalp: when it was finished (the king) said "what do you call the tumour?" I said, "a steatoma, Sir", then, said he, "I hope it will stay at home and not annoy me anymore".
Astley Paston Cooper, 1768-1841

2 To King Edward VII who wanted to postpone his operation for appendicitis: "then Sir, you will go as a corpse".
Frederick Treves, 1853-1923

3 I hope my surgeon is a republican.
Ronald Reagan

4 On President Eisenhower's operation for regional enteritis: the criticism of the operation multiplied in direct ratio to the distance of the critics from the operating room and from the patient.
Leonard Heaton, 1902-1983

Skin is the best

dressing.

Joseph Lister,

1827-1912

Chapter 93

Wounds

1   The wise physician skilled our wounds to heal is more than armies for the common weal.

Homer, 1050-850 BC

2   No wounds should be moistened with anything except wine unless the wound is in a joint. Because dryness is more nearly a condition of health, and moisture more nearly allied to disease.

Hippocrates, 460-377 BC

3   Indeed, above all else, a wound must be made clean.

Theodoric, 1205-1296

4   For it is not necessary... as all modern surgeons profess, that pus should be generated in wounds. Such a practice is indeed to hinder nature, to prolong the disease, and to prevent the conglutination and consolidation of the wound.

Theodoric, 1205-1296

5   Others soak the gauze in water or vinegar ... I always use the blood of the wound for the dressing and have always found myself well served.

Jean Yperman, 1260-1310

6   The wound surgeon: he should always give industrious attention to the parts of the body and their action, and to the blood vessels, so that he may cut, cauterize with corrosives, or burn with iron or gold instruments, without doing injury to the limb.

Hans von Gersdorff, 1480-1540

7   Keep them as neat and clean as possible, and disturb them as little as you can; so far as may be practicable, exclude the air; favor healing under the scab; and ... feed him as you would a woman recovering from her confinement.

Felix Wurtz, 1518-1574

8   I dressed him and God healed him.

Ambroise Paré, 1510-1590

9   Wounds cannot be cured without searching.

Francis Bacon, 1561-1626

10 And yet, how many infallible healing balsams, and wonderful nostrums have been and still are imposed upon the world, not only by Quacks and Empiricks, but too many, whose education and knowledge of the animal oeconomy should render them incapable of low artifact, or ignorance of nature's admirable efforts for her own relief.

John Jones, 1729-1791

11 No wound, let it be ever so small, should be made larger, excepting when preparatory to something else ... it should not be opened because it is a wound but because there is something necessary to be done, which cannot be executed unless the wound is enlarged.

John Hunter, 1728-1793

12 Clinical experience has demonstrated the great value of absorbent material. Discharges drain through them so rapidly that wounds are kept clean and the surrounding parts dry.

Jospeh S Gamgee, 1828-1886

13 The irritation of wound by antiseptic irrigation and washing may therefore now be avoided, and nature left quite undisturbed to carry out her best methods of repair.

Joseph Lister, 1827-1912

14 Skin is the best dressing.

Joseph Lister, 1827-1912

15 Soap and water and common sense are the best disinfectants.

William Osler, 1849-1919

16 The severity of wound infections is merely the result of the extensive destruction of tissues by the projectile ... if it were possible for the surgeon to remove this dead tissue I am sure infections would sink into insignificance.

Alexander Fleming, 1881-1955

17 The great ignominy to the plastic surgeon is his inability to remove a scar without leaving another.

Harold Gillies, 1882-1960, & Ralph D Millard, Jr.

18 When in doubt as to which disinfectant to use, try soap and water.

Martin H Fischer, 1879-1962

19 One of them ... with a compound fracture of the leg, died the next day, the indication of the lethal nature of wounds received on the richly manured grounds of northern France and Flanders.

Geoffrey Keynes, 1887-1982

20   We soon learned ... of the difference between wounds sustained on the clean South African veldt and those contaminated by European mud. Anaerobic bacteria lurking in the soil were responsible for the gas gangrene, which proved to be one of the chief causes of death among those men who reached a base hospital alive.

Geoffrey Keynes, 1887-1982

21   The likelihood of wound infections has been determined by the time the last stitch is inserted in the wound.

Mark M Ravitch, 1910-1989

22   Dressings on undrained wounds serve only to hide the wound, interfere with examination, and to invite adhesive tape dermatitis.

Mark M Ravitch, 1910-1989

23   A surgeon should not wear a long tie that could dangle embarrassingly and dangerously down into a wound or incision while he leans over the patient.

Francis D Moore, 1913-2001

24   The wound is a window into the body.

From the editor

◆   The fate of the surgical wound is sealed during the operation; almost nothing can be done after the operation to modify the wound's outcome.

Take two squirrels, knock their heads together, and if one of them gets a headache, write a paper.

Robert M Zollinger, 1903-1992

Chapter 94

Writing & Publishing

1 Various advantages result even from the publication of opinions; for though we are liable to errors in forming them, yet their promulgation, by exciting investigations and pointing out the deficiencies of our information, cannot be otherwise than useful in the promotion of our science.
John Abernethy, 1764-1831

2 It is a most gratifying sign of the rapid progress of our time that our best textbooks become antiquated so quickly.
Theodor Billroth, 1829-1894

3 Become familiar not only with teaching but also with writing.
Theodor Billroth, 1829-1894

4 I would never use a long word, even, where a short one would answer the purpose. I know there are professors in this country who ligate arteries. Other surgeons only tie them, and it stops the bleeding just as well.
Oliver Wendell Holmes, 1809-1894

5   There is a vast amount of ... worthless material in the literature of medicine ... nine-tenths, at least, of it becomes worthless, and of no interest within 10 years after the date of its publication, and much of it so when it first appears.

John Shaw Billings, 1838-1913

6   Always note and record the unusual. Keep and compare your observations. Communicate or publish short notes on anything that is striking or new.

William Osler, 1849-1919

7   Some people get credit for using a big word instead of a shorter one, yet every now and then a synonym is used because we forget how to spell the word we want to use.

J Chalmers Da Costa, 1863-1933

8   To write an article of any sort is, to some extent, to reveal ourselves. Hence, even a medical article is, in a sense, something of an autobiography.

J Chalmers Da Costa, 1863-1933

9   The writer of textbooks should have a ready imagination and he should understand the child's mind.

Charles H Mayo, 1865-1939

10   The papers, which merit attention because they bear the name of a single famous individual, are becoming fewer every year. Instead, every other article in the medical press has as many authors as an all-star film has credit titles, and their names are of less significance than the legend "from this Clinic" or "from this Institute".

Harvey Graham, ~1939

11   One of the characteristics that often sets apart a junior member of the staff from his colleagues in a striking fashion is his actual ability to finish and report a piece of work ... it is common to find eager young men who have good ideas, who are industrious, who will look things up in books, but it is the exceptional man who seems to have that last little push that allows him to get it down on a piece of paper in order to get it into press.

Elliot Carr Cutler, 1888-1947

12   The medical journals of this country are flooded, as we all know, with immature and sometimes apparently useless publications, and one is sometimes torn between one's desire to keep it down and to let a pupil have the great value to his personality of publishing something.
Elliot Carr Cutler, 1888-1947

13   A busy and active surgeon cannot set aside days and months for writing as the professional writer can. He always has to make literature secondary to action. And the printed pages which bear his name are for the most part the fruit of hours stolen from sleep.
Max Thorek, 1880-1960

14   Textbooks must be orthodox; monographs should be heterodox. We should only beware of an orthodoxy that is accepted without thought and without question, for that indicates an extinct faith.
William Heneage Ogilvie, 1887-1971

15   A man who writes a book or a man who gives a public lecture is committing his reputation to cold print, or to the ears of critical strangers. He must, above all, be accurate. He cannot give expression to those half-formed ideas that are uppermost in his waking moments, to those dreams that he hopes will one day become realities and shake the world.
William Heneage Ogilvie, 1887-1971

16   If a name is attached to an operation or disease, someone else described it earlier, or the originator misunderstood it, or he has been misquoted, or all three.
Mark M Ravitch,1910-1989

17   The first report of any new operation is rarely unfavorable.
Mark M Ravitch,1910-1989

18   Take two squirrels, knock their heads together, and if one of them gets a headache, write a paper.
Robert M Zollinger, 1903-1992

19　The meaning of this paper is hidden by the way it was written.

Mary Evans

20　It is amazing to note that the same hand that is direct and neat with a scalpel becomes paralytic or dyskinetic with a pen.

Seymour I Schwartz

21　We wish to offer to the young or old surgeon the chance to put words on paper, write and re-write, and re-write again. Surgical literature needs all worthwhile contributions, reports and ideas.

Arthur E Baue

22　Publish your results ... results cannot always be interpreted accurately, but they can always be reported accurately. Someone else may define relevance, or the context, or the meaning of something that you have done better than you.

Donald E Fry

23　Everything has been written but not everything has been read.

Bernard Cristalli

24　Writing a manuscript is like a surgical operation: when you undertake it you have to finish.

Alexander A Artemiev

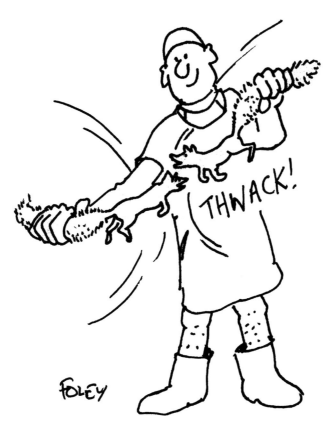

Take two squirrels, knock their heads together,
and if one of them gets a headache, write a paper.

From the editor

◆ Start with case reports. Hemingway started with short stories; only God started with the Bible.

Epilogue

The surgeon of today is not the dramatic individualist that he was. He works more often as one man in a closely-knit team of specialists and research workers. There is much less drama in his individual story. But the story of surgery as a whole is more exacting and more full of promise than ever it was before. And it is a story full of hope that remains always unfinished ...

Harvey Graham, ~1939

Index

Authors

Index

Subject